Learning Disability Policy and Practice

Interagency Working in Health and Social Care
Edited by Jon Glasby

Aimed at students and practitioners, this series provides an introduction to inter-agency working across the health and social care spectrum, bringing together an appreciation of the policy background with a focus on contemporary themes. The books span a wide range of health and social care services and the impact that these have on people's lives, as well as offering insightful accounts of the issues facing professionals in a fast-changing organizational landscape.

Exploring how services and sectors interact and could change further, and the evidence for 'what works', the series is designed to frame debate as well as promote positive ways of interdisciplinary working.

Published titles
French/Swain: *Working with Disabled People in Policy and Practice*
Kellett: *Children's Perspectives on Integrated Services: Every Child Matters in Policy and Practice*
Williams: *Learning Disability Policy and Practice: Changing Lives?*

Forthcoming titles
Baggott: *Public Health and Wellbeing*

Learning Disability Policy and Practice
Changing Lives?

Val Williams

Norah Fry Research Centre at the University of Bristol

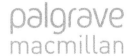

First published 2013 by
PALGRAVE MACMILLAN

Palgrave Macmillan in the UK is an imprint of Macmillan Publishers Limited, registered in England, company number 785998, of Houndmills, Basingstoke, Hampshire RG21 6XS.

Palgrave Macmillan in the US is a division of St Martin's Press LLC, 175 Fifth Avenue, New York, NY 10010.

Palgrave Macmillan is the global academic imprint of the above companies and has companies and representatives throughout the world.

Palgrave® and Macmillan® are registered trademarks in the United States, the United Kingdom, Europe and other countries

ISBN: 978–0–230–57555–4

This book is printed on paper suitable for recycling and made from fully managed and sustained forest sources. Logging, pulping and manufacturing processes are expected to conform to the environmental regulations of the country of origin.

A catalogue record for this book is available from the British Library.

A catalog record for this book is available from the Library of Congress.

10   9   8   7   6   5   4   3   2   1
22   21   20   19   18   17   16   15   14   13

Printed and bound in Great Britain by
CPI Antony Rowe, Chippenham and Eastbourne

To my mother, Denise Puckridge, who gave good
advice on the title for this book

Contents

List of Boxes, Figures and Tables

Boxes

Figure

Tables

Table of Statutes

Acts of Parliament referred to in this book

Adults with Incapacity (Scotland) Act 2000, asp 4
Carers (Equal Opportunities) Act 2004, c. 15
Carers (Recognition and Services) Act 1995, c. 12
Carers and Disabled Children Act 2000, c. 16
Children Act 1989, c. 41
Disability Discrimination Act 1995, c. 50 (revised in 2005)
Disabled Persons Act 1986, c. 33
Education Act 1981, c. 60
Education Act 1993, c. 35
Education Act 1996, c. 56
Education Act 2002, c. 32
Equality Act 2010, c. 15
Health and Social Care Act 2001, c. 15
Human Rights Act, c. 42
Irish Sexual Offences Act 1993
Learning and Skills Act 2000, c. 21
Mental Capacity Act 2005, c. 9
Mental Deficiency Act 1913
NHS Community Care Act 1990, c. 19
Sexual Offences Act 1993, Irish Statute Book
Special Educational Needs and Disability Act, c. 10
Work and Families Act 2006, c. 18

Acknowledgements

Norah Fry Research Centre at the University of Bristol is central to this book, which would never have seen the light of day without the encouragement and contributions of colleagues. I am also really grateful to those who have willingly contributed their expertise, particular research findings or summaries of policy, including Kelley Johnson, who wrote the main part of Chapter 6; and David Abbott, Beth Tarleton, Pauline Heslop, Anna Marriott, Carmel Hand, Ruth Townsley, Marcus Jepson and Sue Porter. My thanks also to others, outside Norah Fry, who have given time and support, including Lesley Russ and Steve Strong. The series editor, Jon Glasby, has continually offered enthusiastic and understanding comments, and the book has also gained greatly from the anonymous reviewers of a previous rather inadequate version.

The comments and experiences of many people with learning disabilities and their families are reflected in these pages; too many to mention all of them individually. However, what really brought the book to life were the contributions of Julian Goodwin, whose story opens Chapter 1, Kerrie Ford, Lisa Ponting, Mouse England, Florence Turner and Kim Norman. They have boldly and honestly talked about their own lives in these pages, and the book would not be possible without them. Thank you all.

A note on terminology

The words 'people with learning disabilities' are used in this book, following the official UK terminology. A full explanation of terms and meanings is given in Chapter 2.

1 Introduction and Overview

This book is about the impact of policy on the lives of people with learning disabilities, and so the best place to start is by listening directly to the account of someone who has experience of the label 'learning disability'. Julian Goodwin here gives a brief overview of some of the important moments in his own life.

" Voice of Experience

My life: by Julian Goodwin

First school

When I was a kid, I went to a mixed school, some boys and some girls. It was a special school for children with disabilities. That was the only school I went to. The girls' dorm was next door, and we kept tapping on the walls, and they used to crawl in. We had a disco at school, I always liked discos. I've always liked to meet new friends, and have friendships. What I didn't like about school was having to stay in the boarding school when my mum and dad went on holiday. The beds were down in a line, it's like being in hospital or something – and they were steel beds, which I didn't like.

When I was a child, I liked listening to Heavy Metal music, which I still do. I like all music, except classical. I had loads of friends. Most of them were from school. And one lived in a big house, and I went to visit. In a boarding school, you do make lots of friends. Whilst I was there, I kept up with them – but as soon as I moved away from school, I didn't keep up. I didn't learn much that was useful to me. Most of the schools were not as good as they are now.

America

When I was a teenager, my dad was head hunted – he was approached by someone in America, to run a Candy Company – a sweet factory. They wanted him to be the vice president. That's why we went over to live in America. I liked the idea, and wanted to go. I think I saw pictures of America, and I imagined it would be hot, which was right. I was about 18.

At first, I went to school in America. It was a mainstream high school. There were lots of new things to learn. When you live in England, you've got to learn English money. But when you move to America, you've got their money to learn. At high school, you've got three floors to use, and a lot more people to try and work around. But I had the scooter then. I had no problem getting around. You did get support in high school, and it was quite easy really, if you didn't understand something, you just asked the teacher. I got on very well with the other kids, and I made some friends there as well.

I see myself as not having a disability, even though I walk on sticks. I can get around OK. Here in England, I went to a special boarding school, but in America, I went to a high school, with regular students. That compared very well with my boarding school. That was smaller, and the high school was a lot bigger. You have more places to explore. Also, you started early and finished school earlier. I set off at 8.30 and I was home by 1.00.

I can remember the graduation where we all had to wear a cap and gown. That's just like here at the University, the only difference is that there when you graduate you take your hat off and chuck it up in the air. And also, what you do there is to have an all-night party, like a gigantic disco.

Making choices in my life

People did talk to me about choices, when I was leaving high school. And I said I'd like to go into the workshop, Lamb's Farm it was called. It was a big industrial place, packeting stuff like medical things. But there weren't any other choices, it was just the one choice, I seem to remember. I felt quite happy because we went on day trips, and they had a block of houses where (if you wanted to) you could stay over. But I used to go home every day. They had their own lake. It was like a farm, the whole complex.

And that's where I met my first girlfriend. She was very pretty.

But soon after, there was another choice to make, as my dad died. That was the choice about moving back to England. It was my decision to move back to England, I was getting sick of things in America. Even though I love hot weather, I didn't want to stay there for any longer.

Work and day centres

Back in England, I went to different day centres. For instance, now I go by minibus to the centre, and come home by minibus. But I am thinking very carefully about reducing one of my days. On a Tuesday, I'm not interested, because I stay in on a Tuesday. And I go three days. The other days, I'm not in the centre. Like for instance on Monday I get picked up, and get taken straight to the rugby club for drama. And spend the day there. At the end of the day, about 3.00, the bus picks me up and he does take me to the centre. And then at the centre, I've got to get back on the bus and go home. It's a lot of travelling around.

But since 1999, I have also had a part-time job. I am an information worker at Norah Fry Research Centre, and I go there one day a week. I used to work on *Plain Facts*, which is a magazine for people with learning difficulties to find out about research. Now it's not funded any more, but I still have a job doing 'easy information' work at Norah Fry. I also do some research, and I'm the secretary for the 'Voice' group. My job helps me to see how information should be easy to understand. Sometimes it is not easy, like in local newspapers.

My job is great, I enjoy getting paid. But I also really like being part of the staff team, and seeing all my colleagues at Norah Fry. I do some teaching now as well, and can tell people lots of things about the more recent changes in my life. Read on ...

Living independently

A few years ago, there was a big change in my life, because my mum died very suddenly. I miss her a lot, but now I live on my own in the flat where we had both moved. I had already spoken with my mum about living on my own before she died. That was my decision: I knew in my own mind what I wanted to do. Sometimes decisions are scary. At the start, I sat on the sofa, thinking to myself – 'god what have I done?'. But now, I love it, because I can invite people around when I want.

I have support staff who come in to see me most days, and do things with me. My family used to do things for me. Like cooking, looking after the flat, looking after my money. But now, with my support, we share the jobs. Like I work the microwave, because if I'm not there, standing by the microwave, my support staff would do it all. And I want to do it. So the only thing they do is work the oven.

So I've got more chance to do things for myself, and it's fun. I could have all-night parties, if I wanted to! But I don't want to go down that road.

Support staff

One of the main things with supporters is to know what is happening. I do generally know who's coming through the door, because I get the list. They're always people I know. But on a Saturday, they put someone's name down, and you expect that person. Sometimes, somebody different comes. For me, that's usually all right, I don't mind.

What's my ideal supporter? I feel happy with anyone and everyone. Someone who does a good job, doesn't rush me. I don't like being rushed. I like taking my own time. That's an important thing, not to be rushed. Also, supporters sometimes fuss too much. When I walk to the front door, I sometimes stumble, but I don't fall over, I catch myself. And whoever I open the door to, they reach out to catch me. I think, 'Excuse me, I'm not going to fall over!'

Another issue I've had is that they come in from an agency with nurses' uniforms, these blue shirts with name tags on them, you know. And on Saturdays, I've asked them not to wear them, because I don't like feeling like I'm in a nursing home. They did listen to me, so they don't wear the uniform on Saturdays now.

I used to get a supporter for just half an hour on a Saturday. I did sit down with my supporters and work out a better way. It was better to tag the time on, so I could have a longer time to be able to go out. On the weekdays, the staff come in at 6 and go away at 7, so I have the evening to myself, which is lovely.

On a Saturday, the supporter comes in and says to me: 'What do you want to do today?' and I go: 'I don't know'. The trouble is that it's not always just about my choice. With one person, I've said to her: 'I want to look around some shops'. And she says, 'We've already done that'. People expect me to come out with something new, and to do different things all the time. So now I have a list of things, then I can just look at them, and say: 'I'd like to do this today, this and this'. If I want to do nothing, then the supporters are sometimes OK with that. But, if it's a nice day, we generally go out somewhere. If it's raining, some staff would say 'It's going to rain, so we'll stay in'. I say that's OK, because I want to anyway. So generally we sort it out together.

The future

My goal for the future is to get married. My girlfriend would feel the same way as me, I know. Age doesn't really matter I don't think, she is 26 and I am 42. We take turns now to go to each other's flats at weekends. She is really fun and cheerful. So I feel very positive about my future. If my mum could see me know, she'd be really proud of me.

Purpose and scope of this book

'What is inclusion, and why does it matter?'; 'can the idea of being a citizen really make a difference?' Questions of this nature are often posed, by those who have contact with people with learning disabilities, in their professional, academic or personal lives. The big ideas in government policy can sound like shallow rhetoric, or even be critiqued as being irrelevant to what is needed at grass-roots level by people with learning disabilities. The aim of this book is to promote reflection on some of these key policy concepts, and to critically evaluate each one in relation to the evidence about the lives of people with learning disabilities. The question threading through the book is: what has policy achieved for the lives of people with learning disabilities – what has it done for them?

As this book will suggest, there is an increasing realization that people with learning disabilities should be included as active, contributing citizens in society. Nevertheless, inclusion is a problematic concept, and achieving it can be a difficult struggle for a group of people who in the past were marginalized or excluded from the mainstream. That is why readers will notice throughout the book stories, comments or discussion directly highlighting the voices of people who have learning disabilities. Julian Goodwin, who has kindly supplied the opening story about his own life, is a colleague at Norah Fry Research Centre, where I work. His life story is a good illustration of the sometimes complex links between policy, real life and practice. As his story shows, there have been many changes in policy which have interacted with personal changes in his own life, resulting in a current lifestyle far removed from that which he would have had some twenty years ago. As his life has moved along, he has gained employment, moved house several times, has lost close family members, but (because of new ideas about personalization) has been able to choose a style of life where he has both privacy and autonomy. His own story about that process shows how he has continued to grow, both in his ability to manage his life and his ability to reflect on it. New challenges can provide opportunities for that growth. Thus, it is by continually returning to the evidence of people's own views and their experiences that current policy and practice can best be judged.

The origins of this book also lie in my own background in working with people with learning disabilities for some forty years. Attitudes towards people with learning disabilities have changed considerably over that period, and it would be true to say that as a special educator, I may have been responsive to individual needs in the 1970s, but did not have strong notions or traditions of inclusion, rights, or autonomy on which to draw. These themes have emerged through new societal discourses related to individual rights, along with thinking about disability based on the social model, which is introduced in Chapter 2. Significantly, the main catalysts for change have been disabled people themselves, rather than non-disabled professionals or policy makers. To some extent, then, policy reflects those major changes in society, and the ideas discussed within the disabled people's movement and also by people with learning disabilities and their families. This book takes the view that policy is not just a 'top-down' notion, but something which emerges from a dialogue between disabled people and government, and that disabled people can have power to make changes for themselves. That idea is sometimes called 'co-production' (Hunter and Ritchie, 2007).

Readers of this book will include all those concerned with the lives of people with learning disabilities. The book is particularly for students in social sciences, or on vocational degrees, aimed at particular professions in social work, direct support or ancillary professions. It is intended to be useful both for those on generic social work programmes, as well as students intending to specialize in Learning Disability, and those on Masters or research-related courses. They will find, however, that it does not lay down the fundamentals of medical or impairment-based knowledge about 'learning disability'; readers should turn elsewhere for that. There are also many other publications which cover extremely well the wide field of study which underpins practice in Learning Disability. Like most of these texts, the current book is rooted in social understandings of what it means to have a learning disability in twenty-first century society. Similarly, Grant *et al.* (2010) adopt a life-cycle approach to Learning Disability, in the light of the English *Valuing People* policy, while Welshman and Walmsley (2006) offer a critical appraisal of community care in perspective, questioning the tension between care and citizenship. Some of the ideas in both these books are reflected in the current volume. Another very useful textbook for those new to the field, at any level, is the collection of edited chapters by Atherton and Crickmore (2011). The current book builds on those volumes, but aims to offer something distinctive, namely an analysis of policy concepts in the light of systematic research evidence about particular areas of life for people with learning disabilities. Those who are called upon to analyse policies, to translate them into practice, and to base all this on evidence, will find material to provide the basis for reflection. The type of discussion provoked will fuel debate for Masters and research students, as well as practitioners, families and, it is hoped, for mixed audiences – anyone who works with or is allied to people with learning disabilities, and for people with learning disabilities themselves. Although it is not an 'easy-read' book, there are key points in each chapter which aim to be more accessible to the general reader, including some people with learning disabilities. Julian Goodwin, whose story opens this chapter, helped to write and check the key points throughout the book.

The purpose of this book is to explore policies and practices in the UK, with particular reference to England and Wales. Examples are frequently offered from Northern Ireland and Scotland, although these are sometimes based on slight variants of the English policies. That is why the term 'learning disability' is used in this book, since that is the term adopted by the UK governments. 'Learning disability' is synonymous with the term 'intellectual disability', used at an international level, and with many other country-specific terms (see Chapter 2. Research or practice is also included at an international level, particularly from Australia, Canada, Iceland and other European countries. Additionally, some chapters look beyond the so-called 'developed' nations of the world, in order to find contrasts and questions to the very philosophy which underpins so much of Western thought. For instance, individual autonomy is not necessarily the most highly prized goal in African countries, and their notions of collectivity and social belonging can contribute positively to the policy debates in the UK.

Disability studies and learning disability

Over the time that Julian Goodwin (in the opening story) has worked at Norah Fry Research Centre, the focus of research at the centre has shifted from being just about 'learning disability'. Most of the research carried out at Norah Fry is now more widely related to disabled people generally, and indeed to the emerging discipline of 'disability studies' (Barnes and Mercer, 2003; Goodley, 2011). The Society for Disability Studies offers the following as part of the defining features of disability studies programmes:

> Disability sits at the center of many overlapping disciplines in the humanities, sciences, and social sciences. Programs in Disability Studies should encourage a curriculum that allows students, activists, teachers, artists, practitioners, and researchers to engage the subject matter from various disciplinary perspectives.
>
> It should challenge the view of disability as an individual deficit or defect that can be remedied solely through medical intervention or rehabilitation by 'experts' and other service providers. Rather, a program in disability studies should explore models and theories that examine social, political, cultural, and economic factors that define disability and help determine personal and collective responses to difference. (Society for Disability Studies, 2012)

The current book sits firmly within that framework. Although the focus is on the lives of people with learning disabilities, the policies which affect their lives are essentially driven by the same goals as for all disabled people. It is by openly examining these policy concepts that the difficulties, tensions and issues for people with learning disabilities can be revealed.

'Disability studies' is driven by a desire for equality, rooted in a human rights approach to disability. Underpinning disability studies is the position that the lives of disabled people are shaped by society in ways that constitute oppression. Throughout this book there is therefore an interest in understanding and critiquing this disablism, in the same way as black scholars are interested in challenging racism. By contrast with previous formulations of disability, which constructed disabled people as individual victims of their impairments, disability studies generally follows the insights of disabled academics, who have observed how the systems and structures of a society favour non-disabled people. These ideas about the social model of disability, and its critiques, are mentioned in Chapter 2, and will be returned to as a basis for thinking about different policy and practice ideas throughout the book. As Goodley (2011) maintains, 'by viewing disability as a cultural and political phenomenon we ask serious questions about the social world'.

The gulf between policy and practice

Although this book aims to mount a critique of some key policy concepts, that does not just mean being 'critical'. On the whole, it will adopt a positive stance, first with an attempt to really understand what each policy concept means; and then to reflect on it in the light of research evidence about people's lives. Each chapter will also offer some deliberately positive, practice-based ideas for putting policy into action. However, there are often some underlying tensions and dilemmas in translating policy into practice, and it is important to unravel some of the competing drivers in public services and supports. The notion of 'autonomy' (see Chapter 8) is a good instance, stemming as it does both from neo-liberal political regimes, but also from the demands of disabled people themselves. However, when applied to people with learning disabilities, it competes with the drive to safeguard and protect people from possible risks and abuse. Instead of rejecting the original idea of autonomy, however, it may be possible to reshape the notion, so that it includes the safeguards provided by collective decision making.

This book has adopted the strategy of focusing on a key policy theme in each of the substantive chapters, in order to link that theme with a particular area of the lives of people with learning disabilities. Each chapter starts with an overview and rationale, and then a discussion of the core policy concept in that chapter, to explain its origins, why it is a major focus for policy, how it relates to Learning Disability, and also how it may be critiqued. Often, that discussion involves a rethink of the term in question and an acknowledgement of its origin, its blurred boundaries and tensions; essentially this book is interested in taking each of the policy concepts in turn, to examine them in the light of the evidence about people's lives. Have these ideas, to date, achieved what policy makers hoped for? For instance, can ideas about human rights help to create better health services for people with learning disabilities? How far have concepts of 'inclusion' influenced the educational experiences of children with learning disabilities, and do parents and families actually benefit from 'partnership working'? As readers might suspect, the evidence is not always positive. Inclusion has been a long time coming in UK schools, and it is well known that people with learning disabilities die prematurely, of preventable illnesses (Mencap, 2007, 2012). Hearing negative examples can cause some people to reject the ideas of 'inclusion' or 'rights' as mere policy rhetoric, and that is a very understandable reaction. Sometimes the ingredients of policy forums seem very far removed from the real lives of people with learning disabilities. This book primarily takes the view that analysis and reflection can help to understand better what these key terms could mean for practice. Progressive and empowering concepts, such as 'autonomy' or 'equality' need to be reflected on and understood as thoroughly as possible, so that they can have a real relationship with practices, and can help to promote debate and reflection. That is the main aim in each chapter of this book.

The structure of each chapter

The chapters are each organized according to a common structure, starting with key points to introduce the content in a more accessible way, and then a rationale to introduce the chapter. The main policy concept is then outlined and discussed, followed by a section to explore and summarize some of the research evidence in the field. Finally, the policy concept is revisited, by examples from practice. The major goal here is to measure the extent to which each policy idea can produce real action for change, and to suggest some ways forward for practitioners. Therefore, while the research evidence is often discouraging or, at best, mixed, in reporting the outcomes for people with learning disabilities, the practice section has a deliberately positive slant. The concluding section of each chapter then reflects on the original policy theme, to outline and remind readers of the tensions and debates which have been raised. As policy is traced into practice and into lived experience, inevitably more questions emerge, and the goal of this book is to provoke debate. Therefore some specific points for reflection are included at the end of each chapter, before a final section to encourage readers to explore further resources. The book as a whole aims to provide enough discussion in order to stimulate critical debate, but also to push each theme to its limits, in suggesting practical solutions.

There are several different types of evidence within this book, but primarily the central part of each chapter focuses on a summary of research evidence from the UK about the particular topic in question. There are also occasional comparisons with other countries, but where they are not explicitly referenced, it can be assumed that the policy arguments are based on social and health care policies in England and Wales. Since the book originates from the Norah Fry Research Centre in Bristol, naturally the research carried out there has a privileged place; however, there is a wide range of research literature in each of the topics under review, and several chapters benefited from the systematic review we carried out in 2008 for a national scoping study about research priorities (Williams *et al.*, 2008).

People with learning disabilities can and do take part in the development of new ideas about their own lives. Where someone's views are directly quoted, that is indicated in the text by a 'Voice of Experience' box. Some of these boxes are from published works, and some from comments or interviews given for the current book. Involvement of people with learning disabilities has been at the forefront of research carried out at Norah Fry Research Centre, and elsewhere in the UK, Ireland, Australia and other countries in Europe, over the past twenty years or more. Therefore, wherever possible, evidence explored about people's lives includes projects where the voices of people with learning disabilities are foregrounded. In some of this work, people occupied the position of co-researcher or self-advocate researcher (Ponting *et al.*, 2010; Townson *et al.*, 2007), while in other studies, people took part by helping to formulate research instruments and collect data (Emerson *et al.*, 2005). This book is not a text book *about* the processes of inclusive research (see Walmsley and Johnson, 2003). Nevertheless, many of the issues and tensions underpinning inclusive research practices are evident in the debates about policy throughout the book. If people with learning disabilities have essentially the same human rights as everyone else, then that should include the right to information about research, and the right to have a say in knowledge about their own position and experience in society. Including people's voices in research, as elsewhere, is often a matter of getting the support right, facilitating without overpowering, and drawing on the collective strength of the self-advocacy movement. All these factors are also important in other areas of practice, and Chapter 10 in particular discusses the central notion of citizenship and participation through the collective movement of people with learning disabilities.

Route map through the chapters

Chapter 2 opens the main part of this book, by introducing and putting down some markers about some central themes that will underpin the whole book. The question of definition of 'learning disability' is an important one, raising as it does the idea of a wide spectrum of individuals, and the significance of diagnosis and labelling. Similarly, the history of learning disability services is referred to briefly, in order to set the context for policies in the twenty-first century. In particular the current policies of personalization are outlined, together with some information about the move to personal budgets in the UK. The collective voice of people with learning disabilities is also a theme, and the notion of 'self-advocacy' is mentioned briefly here. All of these issues will be referred to throughout the rest of the book.

The theme of human rights is developed in Chapter 3, with the main link to health services and access to health care for people with learning disabilities. This chapter strikes at the very right to life itself, which can be undermined if health services do not recognize the needs and value of the lives of patients with learning disabilities. Access to health services is thus an important starting point, with renewed research interest in this area in the UK in 2012.

Chapter 4 follows with a focus on the policy concept of 'inclusion', applying this notion to the field of education. Including disabled children in education is all too often viewed as the insertion of someone with particular needs into an unchanging, unresponsive system. Inclusion however has a wider meaning than that; an inclusive society is one in which all members are valued and have a place. Schools can in some respects be seen as microcosms of society, and so reflecting on 'inclusion' in this context is vital. Despite continued government policy initiatives in the UK, inclusive education still has its problems as well as its successes.

The topic of Chapter 5 is partnership, a key policy word over the past decades. In this context, it will be examined in relation to the families of people with learning disabilities, who, above all, have the right to be considered and treated as equal partners. Their contribution in most countries of the world is indispensable to successful support for people with learning disabilities, of all ages, but there are some profound tensions which still stand in the way of genuine partnership working.

The presence and voice of family carers can be felt throughout the book, not just in Chapter 5, and their central relationship with people with learning disabilities is also one of the key areas for Chapter 6.

Chapter 6 looks at relationships and sexuality. The policy concept chosen in this chapter is 'identity', since it is argued that a loving relationship which is central to one's life profoundly affects a person's sense of identity. Similarly, taking up a role as a parent, or a sexual partner, can often challenge the way other people view a person with learning disabilities.

The sense of personal challenge present in the ideas of sexual identity, presented in Chapter 6, is further explored in Chapter 7 in relation to the period of transition in people's lives. The chapter focuses on people with learning disabilities, who face many transitions, but the particular focus here is on the period of transition to 'adulthood', which is often experienced by families and by young people as 'hurtling into a void'. Nevertheless, the tools of person–centred planning explored in this chapter provide a link with policy, and make it more possible to deliver young people's own goals.

There is a definite link here between policy and practice, as there is also in Chapter 8.

In Chapter 8 we turn to the notion of 'autonomy', which underpins so much of this book. However, this chapter examines the notion of autonomy critically in the light of the Mental Capacity Act 2005 in England and Wales, and the distinction it draws between those who can make decisions with support, and those for whom a best-interests decision may need to be made. In the light of evidence about housing options and living arrangements, these matters are very current in the UK today. The actual lives of people with learning disabilities are affected not just by *where* they live, as has been observed by repeated studies, but also by *how* they are supported.

Chapter **9** turns to the skills of direct support staff, basing the discussion on the notion of 'control', as it is achieved through interactions between support workers and people with learning disabilities. All too often, these relationships are based on a power differential in favour of support workers, and people with learning disabilities themselves say that they want support which is less 'bossy' and more empowering. Chapter 9 touches on some ways of examining and improving direct support practices by filming and discussing natural exchanges between people and their support workers.

The final chapter explores an overarching concept which brings together many of the themes in previous chapters, namely the notion of 'citizenship'. People with learning disabilities, like others in society, are contributors as well as service users. Nevertheless, the idea of being a citizen can also pose problems, when citizenship is something which has to be earned, rather than granted as a social right. Theories of citizenship are therefore useful to examine, in the light of community presence, employment and the direct participation of people with learning disabilities in helping to shape policies and practice.

Readers interested in one area of the lives of people with learning disabilities will no doubt turn to that particular chapter first, and/or consult the index. It is hoped, however, that the idea of exploring policy concepts in practice will lead to

more reflection and debate, with no doubt many competing ideas and issues arising from that reflection. The policy concept for each chapter will be found to
have multiple links, not only with the topic in question, but also in the other areas
of life explored in different chapters. Throughout the book, specific information
from policies or practices is highlighted in boxes, and the comments and stories
of people with learning disabilities are shown in 'Voice of Experience' boxes,
below (see also Julian Goodwin's narrative, above). Their words tend to bring the
ideas of policy and practice to life, and so this introduction will finish with a
central idea of one of our colleagues who has a learning disability:

Voice of Experience

Inclusion is important – everybody I think in the long run whether they have got a
disability or not needs support don't they? When we've got a disability it makes it more
of an issue. I suppose that we need more support than other people, but I just wish
that the people of the ordinary minority would treat people with disabilities with
respect. That's how we want to be included.

Source: Kerrie Ford, 2007

2 | People with Learning Disabilities

Who are people with learning disabilities? In order to explore that deceptively simple question, this chapter will set out some of the starting points, with some underlying ideas and definitions. It will also offer brief outlines of important societal trends, such as personalization and self-advocacy, which provide reference points for many of the other chapters. Although they will be familiar to many readers, it is important to clarify them for those new to people with learning disabilities, or to the UK scene. They are the backdrop for the book as a whole, and the key points in this chapter are listed below:

Key points summary:

- People with learning disabilities face many barriers in society.
- It is hard to know who has a learning disability, even for those who have the label themselves. There are also many different words used in other countries for the same label.
- Some people in the past did not want people with learning disabilities to live. People were also sent away to institutions.
- Now it is different, and all disabled people in the UK should have choice and control over their own support services. That is called personalization.
- Self-advocacy is important. People with learning disabilities can speak up for themselves and help to change things for the better.

The social model and people with learning disabilities

This book follows disabled people themselves, who have reformulated the problems of disability. Instead of focusing on individual impairment, they see disability as created by a society that fails to encompass the range of individual differences of all its members (Oliver, 1990, 2004; Finkelstein, 2004). The social model of disability frames disability as oppression, and attempts to identify and dismantle the barriers that oppress disabled people. Although there has been considerable debate and critique of the social model of disability (Thomas, 2004; Goodley, 2011), arguing for the consideration of impairment alongside social barriers, nevertheless the social model is fundamental, since it stems from disabled people's frustrations and sense of injustice. They reject approaches which focus on 'what is wrong' with the person, and challenge people instead to look at ways of changing the way society as a whole is organized, and the way in which it relates to disabled people. The social model of disability has had a far-reaching and profound influence on policy, and in many ways it underpins and gives rise to all the policy themes in the current book, ranging from human rights and inclusion through to citizenship. As Oliver (2004) has argued, the social model can be criticized and discussed, but essentially it is a tool for change. As such, it offers the most important way of challenging prevailing practice, and repositioning disabled people centre stage. It will be returned to throughout this book.

The impairment of 'learning disability' in particular has traditionally been approached as something that is 'wrong' with the person. Naturally, people with learning disabilities do have health care needs, and impairment-related conditions such as epilepsy may cause significant enduring health problems for many. These issues will be explored further in Chapter 3. However, it must be continually remembered that learning disability in itself is not a medical condition, and nor is it even a collection of individual medical conditions (as is summed up by the title of Rioux and Bach's 1994 book, *Disability Is Not Measles*).

This book will offer many examples of restrictions posed by society, and also other problems, concerns and in fact abusive situations, that face people with learning disabilities in so many areas of their lives. It is easy enough to find such examples. For instance, just as surely as people who use wheelchairs may be physically excluded (by lack of accessible toilets, ramps and lifts) so also people with learning disabilities are excluded by a society that is premised on the ability of all its citizens (Johnson *et al.*, 2010). The barriers people face therefore relate primarily to attitudes of other people, and the lack of ordinary opportunities to live a fulfilled life. This can include barriers in the areas of education, relationships, housing, leisure and employment. For instance, it is still extremely rare for people with a learning disability in Western cultures to have paid employment (Beyer *et al.*, 2004) because economies depend on increasing levels of skill at work (Goodley and Nourouzi, 2005). Therefore, the social model of disability is a strong and useful tool with which to approach the issues facing people with learning disabilities.

   Voice of Experience

Disabling barriers that I face

I want to choose where I live, but I can't. People tell me I cannot move to another town, because I won't be able to get support. This is a barrier about the way support services are organized.

I want to have a job, but I can't read the job adverts. I know I'll also have problems at interviews, and in writing my own CV. People say if I can't do these things, then I wouldn't be able to work.

> **I want to have a close relationship**, but my support staff say it's not safe for me to live with my boyfriend. They think we'll have sex, and that I'll get pregnant. They don't want to be responsible for that.
>
> **I want to have control over my own money** but my family says that I wouldn't be able to manage this. They think I'll spend it all.
>
> **I want to be able to go out, relax and enjoy myself** but I can't because people call me names and make fun of me. They tell me to just ignore this, but it doesn't feel nice. I don't want to go out any more.
>
> Co-tutor with learning disabilities

This range of disabling barriers was mentioned by a person labelled as having a 'learning disability', who was presenting her views to a group of students at the University of Bristol. Many of the barriers she faced seem to come down to people, their reactions, their controlling behaviour – and also possibly harassment and abuse. However, there were also structural problems for her because of the way in which society is organized; for instance, job applications depend on interviews and literacy skills, and support services are organized in local areas, with funds held by them. It can be appreciated from this how social barriers interact with impairment-related barriers, such as lack of ability to read, and possibly also ability to manage one's own money safely. That interrelationship will be a key theme in this book.

Who has a learning disability?

 Voice of Experience

> The words 'learning difficulty' [sic: or 'disability'] were given to us by other people – by those people who diagnosed us. We know we've got this problem, seeing, speaking, understanding – but it doesn't mean we have to have this label on our forehead. I feel like screaming, because people laugh.
>
> *Source*: Self-advocate, in Williams, 2002: 1

Many people reading this book will have a person with learning disabilities in their extended family, others in their immediate family circle. As Julian Goodwin observed at the start of Chapter 1, people do not always identify as having a 'learning disability or difficulty'. The dominant aspect of impairment might differ in school, as compared with post-school settings. Within this shifting and context-dependent perspective, is it possible to know precisely who has a learning disability?

Traditionally, the notion of intelligence testing has underpinned the diagnosis of a learning disability (see Fredrickson and Cline, 2002: 232–45), with norm-based tests yielding an intelligence quotient (IQ). Thus the category of 'severe learning disability' is notionally associated with an IQ of below 50, and a moderate learning disability with an IQ of between 50 and 69. However, there have been many issues raised about the validity of IQ tests, and in fact their usefulness, depending as they do on a fixed notion of general intelligence. In practice, individual people with learning disabilities have different profiles of skills. The current definition of 'learning disability' in England was written into the national strategy *Valuing People* in 2001, and is given in Box 2.1.

Box 2.1	Definition of 'learning disability'

This has been the English definition of learning disability since 2001:

- a significantly reduced ability to understand new or complex information, to learn new skills
- a reduced ability to cope independently
- which started before adulthood, and with a lasting effect on development.

Source: DH, 2001

The enduring tension, reflected in the above definition, is whether to define the person, the level of support needed, or some interaction between the two. There is clearly some circularity if people are defined entirely by the types of support they get, as they may well over time become more able to 'cope independently' and understand new information. The risk is then that they are no longer considered as having a disability, and may qualify for less (or no) support services. There seem to be three underlying reasons for definitions:

1. To match an individual to a particular service, by virtue of their particular characteristics and needs.
2. To exclude other people from that service or that category.
3. To aid our understanding of how to support people.

Taking these positions in turn, first it is clear that the usefulness of a definition is related very much to the specific services offered, the demands on the individual, and thus to the context. As Chapter 4 will discuss, for instance, the definition of 'learning difficulty' in education in the UK relates to the level of support required to access the curriculum. The second point about definitions is that they both include, and specifically serve to exclude, certain individuals. For instance, definitions such as the English one above are intended to identify a category of people with more pervasive learning disabilities, and to exclude groups such as those with dyslexia or with acquired brain injury. This might seem a logical goal, since the causes and outcomes may be quite different. However, the third point about practical support is perhaps the most important for the current book. Definitions are useful, only if and when they serve to delineate a group of people who can be supported or helped in specific ways by specific services.

Consider the examples below, which are stories based on research evidence:

Examples of people being defined in relation to services

- A man called Ben lived alone, but had 24-hour support (i.e. a support worker was always with him). This cost a lot of money, and so the local authority tried to redefine him as someone with 'moderate learning disabilities' (instead of severe learning disabilities). This would imply that he did not need the intensive support he was currently given. Ben's family was naturally upset by this change in the use of language!
- A general practitioner (family doctor: GP) in the south-west of England felt that he treated all his patients in the same way. However, a family complained to him that they were unable to bring their son for a consultation, since his level of frustration meant that he could not wait for long in the waiting room. In order to access health services, he needed a small amount of special consideration. This led the GP to work out how many patients with learning disabilities, and family carers, he had on his list. His service could only improve if he had a way of defining who was who.

A key question to consider is whether to focus on the individual impairment, or the way in which that person's problems are produced by society. For instance, despite the fact that *Valuing People* (DH, 2001) explicitly adheres to a social understanding of the barriers faced by people with learning disabilities, it will be seen that the English definition of 'learning disability' given above is very much rooted in medical understandings. The definition assumes that one can assign the label 'learning disability' to people because of the fact that they *cannot* perform functionally ('a reduced ability to cope independently') and that this lack of functional ability is connected to their brains ('a significantly reduced ability to understand new or complex information'). Moreover, the definition assumes the unchanging nature of learning disability; this is something 'which started before adulthood' and has a 'lasting effect' on development. By contrast, many would argue that a learning disability is a social construct of particular societies, and is thus both culturally relative and produced by particular social practices (Rapley, 2004). Whatever the case, the label 'learning disability' carries with it a diagnosis of difference, and implications that people's cognitive capacity is limited. This raises some profound dilemmas, in relation to the themes of this book. Can a person with learning disabilities actually perform as an autonomous member of society, with the rights and responsibilities of a full citizen? As Gillman *et al.* (2000) argue, it is a diagnosis that has a pervasive effect on a person's whole being, and is not something that is easily cast aside.

What words should be used to describe people?

Although related to the question of definition, the issue about terminology is conceptually distinct. Terminology in the field of 'Learning Disability' has been prone to changes, broadly tracking the way society's thinking about disabled people has developed. However, across the globe, there are still many different ways of referring to people with learning disabilities, as seen in Table 2.1 below.

Table 2.1	Terminology used to refer to people with learning disabilities

Term used (more than one may be used in each country)	% of countries
Mental retardation	76
Intellectual disabilities	56.8
Mental handicap	39.7
Mental disability	39
Learning disabilities	32.2
Developmental disabilities	22.6
Mental deficiency	17.2
Mental subnormality	11.6

Source: Based on statistics from WHO, 2007

When considering the debates for and against various terms, it is important to take into account:

1. Labelling as power: who is doing the labelling? Doctors, educators, psychologists, social workers? Or, does the label come from the person themselves, signifying solidarity with a group?
2. The social value of the term: some labels are quickly used as insults or abuse, and contribute to the stigma experienced by the individual.
3. How the label affects identity: the label may move others away from seeing the individual as a human being, with unique personality and skills.

The very multiplicity of labels, the differences between people labelled, and the continued debates about terminology remind one that 'learning disability' itself is still a contested concept (Eayrs *et al.*, 1993; Beart *et al.*, 2005). Perhaps this is as it should be. The attempt to grasp the essence of what 'learning disability' might constitute is probably flawed, as it leads back into medical thinking, where it is assumed that everyone with that label has a 'real' and presumably similar, problem in their brain: if labels have to be used, especially in an area as sensitive as learning disability, then the best way to know what words to use is to ask the people to whom the label is applied. In the self-advocacy movement in England, people have always said that they do not want any labels, as was evident in the quotation at the beginning of this chapter. That is the origin of the phrase 'People First'. However, as Sutcliffe and Simons (1994) pointed out, self-advocates said that, if they had to have any label, they would prefer 'learning *difficulty*'. In the early years of the twenty-first century, most have shifted towards the official UK terminology of 'learning disability', although both these terms are used differently in countries such as the USA, where they refer to dyslexia or specific learning difficulties. That is not the sense in which 'learning disability' is used here.

The words 'learning disability' are used in the UK in fact to refer to a very wide range of individuals. People with learning disabilities who have the highest support needs generally require someone on a round-the-clock basis to support them, help them eat, or manage the basics of everyday life (an 'inability to carry out personal care routines'. Many people in these categories will have different ways of communicating, and will not use a fully formed language (whether that is a spoken or a sign language). Without support, they would exercise little or no 'choice or control' over their immediate environment. People defined as having a 'profound or multiple learning disability' (PMLD) (Mencap, 2008) are those who have a range of concurrent impairments, including a profound learning disability; they also have severe communication impairments, and many will have additional sensory or complex health needs.

Another group who come into the 'high support' category are those who have so-called 'severe challenging behaviour'. Without support, they would run the risk of danger to their own life and health (or that of others). The definition of severe challenging behaviour has long been accepted in the UK as the following:

> Severely challenging behaviour refers to culturally abnormal behavior(s) of such an intensity, frequency or duration that the physical safety of the person or others is likely to be placed in serious jeopardy, or behaviour which is likely to seriously limit use of, or result in the person being denied access to, ordinary community facilities. (Emerson, 1995: 4–5)

It is important to note that, although the term 'challenging behaviour' is often applied to individuals, the term was originally intended (Mansell, 2007) to focus attention on the socially constructed, interactional nature of challenging behaviour.

At the other end of the scale, a wider definition of 'learning disability' will include those who do not receive specific services, but may be said to have 'moderate' or 'mild' learning disabilities, since they find some of the tasks of independent living difficult. They may for instance, have problems with budgeting, with managing a family, or with basic literacy skills, without some support. If one includes all these people, there are currently over one million people with learning disabilities in the UK aged 15 and over (Emerson and Hatton, 2004) and this number is set to increase between 2009 and 2026. People with learning disabilities are living longer, and older adults with learning disabilities are understandably costly in terms of their personal care (Strydom et al., 2010; Emerson and Hatton, 2009). While definitions therefore matter, this book will take the view that they should not restrict a person's identity. As people become older, they have many roles and experiences, not just that of being a person with learning disabilities.

Warnings from the past

It was not until the era of industrialization in the nineteenth century (Richardson, 2010) that Western societies were influenced by the expectation of perfection in intelligence and aspiration in the growing middle classes and upper classes. Fuelled by Darwin's ideas about evolution, theories of genetics sprang up which discriminated cruelly against those who were perceived to be different. Not only were people with learning disabilities seen as a threat in terms of their anti-social behaviour, but they were also seen as a threat to the very fabric of society because of their presumed tendency to reproduce more disabled children. Eugenicist ideas reached their culmination in Germany during the time of the Third Reich. Disabled people, and particularly those with learning disabilities, were assumed to contaminate the 'pure race' of Aryans, and they were the first to be exterminated. By contrast with Germany, as Concannon (2005: 16–28) points out, the response in the UK to these eugenicist worries was to incarcerate people in long-stay institutions, far from friends and family and literally out of sight of mainstream society. People with learning disabilities, even today, feel the weight of historical contempt from which they have emerged; whether the response was to kill, to sterilize or to lock away, all these acts were essentially aimed at stopping people with learning disabilities from existing at all, or at least from being visible in society. This was the supreme devaluation.

The origins of a stigmatized identity can thus be witnessed in the historical treatment of people with learning disabilities. In many Western countries, people with learning disabilities, along with 'moral defectives', alcoholics and those with mental health problems, were bracketed together. Moreover, the twentieth century reinforced the fear of those 'excluded' groups in the UK and elsewhere, by advocating their removal from normal society (Atkinson *et al.*, 1997; Richardson, 2010). In the UK, a century ago, this move was underwritten by the Mental Deficiency Act of 1913, which defined four 'classes' of deficiency:

- Idiot: unable to protect themselves from common dangers.
- Imbecile: could protect themselves from common dangers, but unable to take care of themselves.
- Feeble-Minded: required care to protect themselves.
- Moral Defectives: criminal or vicious personalities, including unmarried mothers.

It was this Act which introduced the Board of Control, and which prompted the widespread creation of asylums or institutions where large numbers of 'deficient' people could be housed, away from the mainstream of society.

In the year 2012, there are still many people with learning disabilities alive who are witnesses to institutional life. It is always important to listen to them, and to remember the past, so that the traces of institutional thinking and practices can be recognized and challenged in current practices. Several have contributed to histories (see Atkinson *et al.*, 1999); for instance, a group of people who lived at Hortham Hospital in Bristol, took part in a project in 1994 to write their own history, based on photos from the hospital archive. The points they made about institutional life are given below, with quotations from the book they produced.

> **" Voice of Experience**
>
> - People were not informed why they were 'sent' to institutions ('I didn't know a soul when I went there, and it was quite frightening').
> - Everything took place within the same institution, including schooling ('All the children used to go to the school, and I remember all the children. They're dead now, most of them').
> - The daily routine was fixed in order to suit the staff ('All the wards used to be locked just after 8.00 at night, and all we lot would go to bed just after 7.00').
> - There was overcrowding and no privacy ('You couldn't swing a cat').
> - People who lived in the hospitals did a lot of work, but didn't get any pay ('We made rugs. We sold them, but we never got the money. I don't know where it went').
> - Staff were in control of residents, and appeared to treat the hospital as if it were for their own benefit. This certainly included custodial treatment of residents, if the rules were broken ('Sometimes they stopped your privileges – that meant no money all week. Or they put you in straitjackets, or you got locked up in a punishment room in the dark').
> - Despite all these negative points, people who lived in the institutions clearly had a sense of belonging, and enjoyed certain aspects of group life, including the entertainments and sports ('My friend was in the football team. I was in the cricket team ... more or less to pass the time away').
>
> *Source*: Hortham Memories Group, 1994

Community-based services and normalization

Over the past forty years, de-institutionalization has been a key feature of learning disability policy in the UK, and in many other countries across the globe, including for instance Sweden (Ericsson, 2002) and Australia (Johnson *et al.*, 2005). It was associated with and driven very much by the model of 'normalization', which was highly influential in learning disability services. Originating in Denmark (Nirje, 1970), normalization was quickly taken up in the USA by Wolfensberger (1972) who became its chief proponent. Essentially, it was about an ordinary lifestyle for people with learning disabilities, and emphasized the type of support needed in order to achieve this. It was driven by a humane ideology, that people should be seen and respected as human beings, and was very much a tool to fight back against the dehumanizing aspects of institutional care. In the UK, one of the most important aspects of normalization was the adoption of the 'five accomplishments' by which to measure services (Brown and Smith, 1992) and these are still very relevant today.

Box 2.2   **O'Brien's five accomplishments**

Community presence: the right to take part in community life and to live and spend leisure time with other members of the community.
Relationships: the right to experience valued relationships with non-disabled people.
Choice: the right to make choices, both large and small, in one's life. These include choices about where to live and with whom to live.
Competence: the right to learn new skills and participate in meaningful activities with whatever assistance is required.
Respect: the right to be valued and not treated as a second-class citizen.

Source: based on Brown and Smith, 1992

Since the 1970s and 1980s, there have been many critics of 'normalization' (Walmsley, 1997; Chappell, 2000), particularly since in its later manifestations as 'social role valorization', it seemed to imply that people had to fit into typical social roles in order to be valued by society. With the move towards disability rights, and new ideas about social barriers, this notion of fitting in appeared to be rather weak, and even discriminatory. Nevertheless, the philosophy of normalization had and does have a tremendous impact on service provision, and this book would not want to argue with the idea of the five accomplishments of service provision.

Personalization, choice and control and independent living

Since the early years of the new millennium, the UK government has steadily moved towards a policy known as 'personalization' (DH, 2005, 2006). The idea at the heart of personalization is that individual service users should be able to exercise their own choice and control over their service supports and in fact over their whole life. Building on the former framework for direct payments (DH, 1996), personalization is driven by the need to progress independent living outcomes for all disabled people. It is important to stress here that living independently is effectively synonymous with 'choice and control'. It does not entail living on one's own, nor does it rely on the learning of new skills for independence, as many people with learning disabilities are led to believe. This is the definition of independent living from the Disability Rights Commission:

> All disabled people having the same choice, control and freedom as any other citizen – at home, at work, and as members of the community. This does not necessarily mean disabled people 'doing everything for themselves', but it does mean that any practical assistance people need should be based on their own choices and aspirations. (Morris, 2003: 4)

Independent living, as it is defined here, is about getting the support right. It is about effective planning, rights, inclusion and also about everyday interactions with support staff. Thus the notion of independence with support underpins each chapter in this book.

Local authorities in England and Wales were expected to implement change (DH, 2008a) by 2011, in order to shift social care for disabled and older people towards:

- a more preventative and less crisis-driven mode (DH, 2008a: 4);
- a less bureaucratic and more 'personalised' form of service 'which is on the side of the people needing services and their carers' (DH, 2007: 1); and
- a system which should 'empower citizens to shape their own lives and the services they receive' (PMSU, 2007).

Although this move towards more personalized services is mirrored in several countries (Townsley *et al.*, 2009), the term 'personalization' can be put into practice in different ways. In England and Wales, the major operational tool for delivering personalization is the 'personal budget', which is a term used to describe the way in which social services resources can be managed on an individual basis, according to the assessed needs of each disabled person (Carr, 2010).

The main features of a personal budget system, in theory, are that:

1. Service users should be able to assess their own needs, initially, in order to apply for social support. There is an element here both of empowerment, but also of rationing, since people's eligibility can be questioned at this stage.
2. Once accepted as eligible (see below: Box 2.3), a disabled or older person should be told their indicative budget, which will enable them to plan for their own support needs.
3. People can choose whether to take their personal budget as 'cash' (a direct payment), or to realize it in a number of other ways – including the purchase of services through a support organization, or as a combination of direct payment and directly provided services.
4. Once service users have planned out what will work for them, the social services department has to validate the plan, to ensure that budgets are well spent, and that the service user's outcomes are likely to be met by their plan.
5. Essentially, the next step is simply to put the plan into action, and for the budget then to be monitored on an annual basis by social services.

Research in this field (Glendinning *et al.*, 2008) investigated the possibility that these budgets could be holistic, in the sense that one budget could incorporate the various sources of health, work-related and social care support money that an individual might accrue. That goal has proved elusive, and older people in particular were found to benefit the least from personal budgets. For people with learning disabilities, much depended on the support they had from family and friends, and that has been a constant theme of research since the pilot evaluation.

People with learning disabilities were amongst the first to be supported by an organization called 'In Control' to take up budgets, and to plan for their own social support. However, one of the first dilemmas for them relates back to the very definition of 'learning disability'. As discussed above, it is evident that a 'learning disability' is not a fixed concept. The term is used in ways that are very much dependent on the types of services available, and this will in turn depend on the level of resources that society is willing to spend on this sector. Therefore, people who identify as having a learning disability may not always be eligible for social support in England. The eligibility criteria for the main two 'fundable' or eligible categories of need are given in Box 2.3.

Box 2.3	Fair access to care

A person has critical needs – when (if it were not for the support provided):

■ life is, or will be, threatened; and/or
■ significant health problems have developed or will develop; and/or
■ there is, or will be, little or no choice and control over vital aspects of the immediate environment; and/or
■ serious abuse or neglect has occurred or will occur; and/or
■ there is, or will be, an inability to carry out vital personal care or domestic routines; and/or
■ vital involvement in work, education or learning cannot or will not be sustained; and/or
■ vital social support systems and relationships cannot or will not be sustained; and/or
■ vital family and other social roles and responsibilities cannot or will not be undertaken.

A person has substantial needs – when (if it were not for the support provided):

■ there is, or will be, only partial choice and control over the immediate environment; and/or
■ abuse or neglect has occurred or will occur; and/or
■ there is, or will be, an inability to carry out the majority of personal care or domestic routines; and/or
■ involvement in many aspects of work, education or learning cannot or will not be sustained; and/or
■ the majority of social support systems and relationships cannot or will not be sustained; and/or
■ the majority of family and other social roles and responsibilities cannot or will not be undertaken.

Source: DH, 2003b

New guidance (DH, 2010) is set in the context of a vision for universal, community-based personalized services (DH, 2008), and recognizes that service users will only have choice and control over their own support if timely, preventative and supportive services are provided to those with low levels of need. However, these are not envisaged as needing extra resources, nor as taking away resources from those with the highest level of needs. Instead, there is a new vision of support being available through local community resources, and social services departments are urged to work in partnership with other sectors of the council, through a holistic, whole-system approach.

> Prevention should not be seen as the sole preserve of adult social services or the NHS [National Health Service], rather it is most effective when brought about through partnerships between different parts of a council and between other user and carer-led, voluntary and community organisations. (DH, 2010: 16)

A second major dilemma relates to the ability of people with learning disabilities to actually decide for themselves and to plan and manage the details of their own support. Many would argue, like Dowse (2009), that these neo-liberal aims of policy are by definition impossible for most people with learning disabilities. If they could exercise autonomy, then they would cease to have a learning disability and would also no longer be eligible for services. However, there are other, more nuanced arguments about autonomy with support. As Williams and Porter (2011) found in research for the Office for Disability Issues, people with learning disabilities generally had support from family, person-centred planning approaches (see Chapter 7 in this book) and from other voluntary sector organizations in developing their own support plans and 'taking control'. Duffy (2003) also outlines the possibilities for support, and the various roles that might be necessary on an ongoing basis, for people with learning disabilities to become active citizens and to develop the kinds of support which will suit them best. These matters about personalization will be returned to throughout the book, and represent an underpinning notion about current English social care policy, affecting all disabled people.

Self-advocacy: the voice of people with learning disabilities

While the social model of disability (see above) is the badge of honour of all disabled people, underpinning the international disabled people's movement, people with learning disabilities in the UK have moved along a different but parallel path, in their own self-organization. This may be partly because of the need for support, and the strong role played by 'allies' in the support of their efforts to speak up for their own rights (Goodley, 1997; Williams, 2011: ch. 10).

Through the 1980s and 1990s, people with learning disabilities in the USA and then in the UK took action to form a social movement of their own. This is known as the self-advocacy movement, and includes groups known as 'People

First'. In the self-advocacy movement, people do not only speak up about their own issues, they can define those issues for themselves, and in the process can define themselves too:

> It takes a lot of courage and strength to fight against people who have the power to define who you are. (Souza, 1997: 6)

Some authors (Goodley, 2000; Danforth, 2000) have considered these issues in the context of Foucault's concepts of power and knowledge, and in particular his reference to subjugated voices. Foucault (1980: 81–2) claims that: 'it is through the reappearance of this knowledge, of these local popular knowledges, these disqualified knowledges, that criticism performs its work'. The voices of people with learning disabilities constitute an extreme form of disqualified knowledge, since the dominant social view is that the impairment itself is defined by a lack of ability to represent oneself. The very term 'self-advocacy' is a way of fighting back, and of marking the assumption that these are people who have not previously been able to advocate for themselves, as Goodley points out:

> The term self-advocacy has been applied to account for the self-determination of minority groups who have historically been denied a 'voice' ... the self-determination of people with learning difficulties is emphasised and members of this labelled group are referred to as self-advocates. (2000: 7)

'Self-advocacy' is a term of the oppressed, a political weapon, that people can grasp in order to make their own voices heard.

> Self-advocacy is about independent groups of people with disabilities working together for justice by helping each other take charge of their lives and fight discrimination. (Nellis, 1994: 1)

The UK movement started during the 1980s (Dybwad and Bersani, 1996), and was at first supported by non-disabled partners such as CMH (Campaign for Mental Handicap, now Values into Action) and Mencap. The model for self-advocacy in this country drew largely on the movement already establishing itself in the USA, and statements about this by self-advocates themselves are often included in academic publications (Sutcliffe and Simons, 1994; Goodley, 2000). Self-advocacy assumed particular prominence following the English learning disability strategy, *Valuing People* (DH, 2001). In addition to the personal, individual meanings of self-advocacy, there is a political need for self-advocacy to provide the context for what is often termed 'empowerment' (Ramcharan *et al.*, 1997). If people can represent themselves, then they can be expected to be meaningful partners in government policy making. Additionally, self-advocacy is increasingly referred to as a social movement (Goodley, 2000: 3). By making a parallel with the struggles of other minority groups, such as black people or women, Goodley positions self-advocacy as a collective, political movement which belongs to people with the label of learning disabilities. Authors such as Goodley (1997) and Brechin (1999: 65) express the hope that the control exerted by self-advocates over their own affairs will result in an 'emancipatory politics of identity'. Self-advocacy can completely change the balance of power, by including people meaningfully within the debates concerning their own lives.

There are many questions embedded here about the way in which self-advocates actually speak up and represent issues fairly, and about the extent to which people who have a learning disability can be expected to discuss matters within political arenas. These are taken up in later chapters, particularly in Chapter 10. However, a fundamental point to note is the positioning of the self-advocacy movement within the more general disabled people's movement. In the UK, there has historically been a certain tension between the two movements, with the latter being initially slow to include people with learning disabilities in its ranks (Chappell, 2000). In recent years, that difference is gradually being eroded, and more common connections are emerging between the thinking which underpins both the disabled people's movement and self-advocacy organizations. All are united by a common aim, to combat barriers in society, whether these are physical access problems, or attitudinal barriers. All these groups also have to grapple with the same conceptual problems, continually questioning and trying to redefine what the word 'disability' actually means. One of the aims of the current book is to contribute to that discussion.

Reflection exercises

At the end of each chapter in this book, readers will find suggestions for discussion and reflection. These are intended to demonstrate that the matters discussed in these pages do not offer final answers, and nor are they set in stone. Most of the issues will raise more questions than they solve. Therefore, it is important that readers interact with these pages, to bring their own experiences and knowledge to bear on the questions about how best to support people with learning disabilities.

1. After reading this introductory chapter, it is useful to reflect on the 'lessons from the past', and to find out more about how and why eugenicist philosophy was applied to disabled people. Consider carefully what elements of these attitudes and practices still exist in societies today.

2. The social model has been described (Oliver, 2004) as a tool for change. Does the social model really engage with the issues facing all people with learning disabilities, and is it adequate to ensure that positive changes happen in their lives?

3. Some people reading this book will be practitioners, or those training to enter various professions. After following up some of the

self-advocacy material in this chapter and elsewhere, discuss how your own services work with others to include the voices of people with learning disabilities, and how that element of self-advocacy could be improved.

Suggested further resources

This chapter has only provided a very quick skim over some fundamental issues in the lives of people with learning disabilities, and there are many texts that will give more detail. The history of people with learning disabilities, as well as questions of definition and labelling, are all covered in recent edited collections such as:

1. Grant, G., Goward, P., Richardson, M. and Ramcharan, P. (eds) (2010) *Learning Disability: A Life Cycle Approach*, 2nd edn, Buckingham: Open University Press.

   Moving through from childhood to ageing and end-of-life issues, this volume contains a wealth of useful information from researchers and practitioners about the issues facing people with learning disabilities. It is very good value for money, and would be recommended to anyone new to the field.

2. Atherton, H. and Crickmore, D. (eds) (2011) *Learning Disabilities: Towards Inclusion* 6th edn, London: Churchill Livingstone.

   Formerly edited by Bob Gates, this book provides a good, comprehensive overview of many key issues in the lives of people with learning disabilities. It also has an online version and exercises for each chapter.

3. The *social model of disability* is best explored by picking one of the collections of writings by disabled people who developed that model, such as:

   Barnes, C. and Mercer, G. (eds) (2003) *Disability Policy and Practice: Applying the Social Model of Disability*, Leeds: Disability Press.
   Swain, J., French, S., Barnes, C. and Thomas, C. (eds.) (2004) *Disabling Barriers: Enabling Environments*, 2nd edn, London: Sage.

   There are many critiques and debates about the social model, and these could be accessed for instance in:

   Kristiansen, K., Yehman, S. and Shakespeare, T. (eds) *Arguing about Disability: Philosophical Perspectives*, London: Routledge.

Goodley, D. (2011) *Disability Studies: An Interdisciplinary Introduction*, London: Sage.

4. *Self-advocacy* has also been the topic of books, such as Goodley, D. (2000) *Self-Advocacy in the Lives of People with Learning Difficulties*, Buckingham: Open University Press.

   To get a flavour of self-advocacy groups in the UK, their own websites are good starting points:

   www.peoplefirstltd.com
   www.bsgpf.org.uk

   More examples are given in the resources section in Chapter 10.

5. Readers wishing to find out more about *personalization* can go to the website of the Social Care Institute for Excellence: www.scie.org.uk. Follow the links to 'people with learning disabilities' and then to 'personalization'. A very useful resource is the 'Rough Guide to Personalisation' by Sarah Carr.

   Explanations and stories to bring personalization to life can be found at the In Control website: www.in-control.org.uk

3 Taking a Human Rights Approach to Health

Human rights are fundamental to everything else in this book, and so provide the main policy theme which frames this first substantive chapter. In relation to human rights, the chapter will focus on the issues to do with equal access to general health care for people with learning disabilities in the UK.

Key points summary:

- Everyone has the same human rights, including the right to life. That means that everyone should have the same chance of getting good health care.
- There has been lots of progress in medicine. That has made a big difference for some people with learning disabilities.
- But the way health care is set up may mean that there are barriers for people with learning disabilities to get ordinary treatment. That means that some people die before they should.
- Everyone is responsible for looking after themselves. Doctors and nurses can help people have a healthy life, and so can families, friends and others who support them.
- Thinking about human rights is useful, as it helps to see what is wrong and what could be changed.

Introduction and overview

 Voice of Experience

I went to the GP with my mum, but he only spoke to her. My mum told him not to do that, but I couldn't get my point across at all. I gave up really, because I couldn't understand what was going on.

Source: person with learning disabilities in workshop: Williams *et al.*, 2008b: 45

There have been immense advances in health treatments over the past fifty years, for instance in understanding and tackling the acute problems of cancer and heart disease. These have benefited people with learning disabilities as well as other patients in the UK. There has also been progress in specific medical knowledge and treatment of conditions that particularly affect people with learning disabilities, such as epilepsy, and certain genetic conditions. However, a learning disability is not in itself a health problem, although the label is rooted in cognitive differences. It may therefore seem odd that for many years, learning disability was assumed to be somewhat akin to a disease, which could be diagnosed by medical practitioners (see Rioux and Bach, 1994: page 13 of this book). Nevertheless, people with learning disabilities fall ill, have certain predispositions towards certain health problems, and also need good health advice and treatments, as everyone in the community does.

The aim of this chapter is to consider the evidence about health care advances, as well as the problems, for people with learning disabilities in the UK, and to highlight some of the positive practices that will ensure all patients have their rights to health care met. For instance, the scenario mentioned by a person with learning disabilities in the opening quotation is typical of the problems faced by someone who cannot even understand what the doctor is saying. This group of patients is regularly sidelined, with others taking over responsibility, including family members, support workers or other carers.

This chapter is not just about illness, and coping with illness. It will start with a consideration of human rights statements and instruments, and what they imply about the right to a healthy life. Human rights are an important starting point for any practitioner, since they provide a framework which allows us to see things in a new light, and to question oppressive practices. The following part of the chapter looks at research evidence about the generic lifestyle and social issues which are known to affect people with learning disabilities, and evidence about the barriers and problems in accessing health services. It will also look more closely at what is known about some of the specific issues for a certain group of people, those who are born with multiple and complex physical and sensory problems. There are further groups who also access specialist services by virtue of particular sets of specialist 'needs', namely those who acquire mental health problems, and those who are deemed to have 'challenging behaviour'. For rather different reasons, all these groups may need access to intensive health interventions at certain points in their lives. However, this chapter will focus mainly on how health services can and should operate in a holistic way, treating people as individual human beings, and supporting wherever possible the individual to make decisions about their health. The final part of the chapter will then return to the theme of human rights, to work out what solutions can be put in place, to ensure that the health inequalities faced by people with learning disabilities are redressed.

Key policy concept: human rights

 Voice of Experience

I think of life as a person with learning difficulties as being taken to watch a football match, where life is that football match, and never being allowed to join in. People with learning difficulties have the same dreams, inspirations and aspirations as everyone else but we are held back from engaging in life. If you think of your most cherished moments in life, of the things that you still look back on and smile, I expect it is something that people with learning difficulties would get held back from doing.

Source: Andrew Lee, Director, People First, cited in Joint Committee on Human Rights (2008: 30)

The purpose and origin of human rights statements

The concept of human rights is about valuing human beings as equals. In one sense, the notion of human rights is universal, and does not differentiate. The human rights agenda effectively sets itself to address society's barriers, and sets the standard by which we measure what is happening for *all* citizens, in every country:

> Human rights belong to everyone, and they provide a very important means of protection for disabled people. Human rights place authorities in the UK – including the Government, hospitals and social services – under an obligation to treat you with fairness, equality, dignity and respect. (BIHR, 2006: 6)

However, the notion of 'human rights' is generally invoked specifically in relation to groups of people who might be disadvantaged, either through active discrimination or by the way society's institutions are formulated, without taking account of their needs. If certain groups of people are not valued equally, this is mirrored in the way in which society treats them, denying them opportunities, services or citizenship. For instance, the UK Joint Committee on Human Rights for people with learning disabilities (2008) found that there are many ways in which the lives of people with learning disabilities have not been valued in the same way as those of other human beings. The concept of rights thus lies at the heart of the social model of disability (see Chapter 2, pp. 12–14), which is about the exclusion of disabled people from a society which is formulated around the needs of the non-disabled population. A rights based approach to disability challenges the assumption that disabled people need some type of charity, which is essentially at the generous discretion of benevolent tax payers in society (Campbell and Oliver, 1996).

The idea of setting out explicitly the rights of human beings, in order to ensure justice and equality, has a very long history. For instance, there are statements about rights in both Greek and Roman laws, and in the Magna Carta and of course in the US Declaration of Independence, although all of these had various restrictions in their application. However, human rights statements were revitalized following the atrocities in the Second World War. Human rights lawyers sought to formulate statements of basic rights, to protect the liberty and dignity of all human beings and to prevent crimes against humanity from every being repeated; the Universal Declaration of Human Rights (UN, 1948), adopted by the UN General Assembly on 10 December 1948, was thus framed as a tool, or defensive mechanism, to fight back against the evils of society. Although they are all interconnected, two of the articles detailed in the Universal Declaration might be particularly important to note here, in relation to health and the right to life. Article 3 states that 'everyone has the right to life, liberty and security of person', while Article 25 states that:

> Everyone has the right to a standard of living adequate for the health and well-being of himself and of his family, including food, clothing, housing and medical care and necessary social services, and the right to security in the event of unemployment, sickness, disability, widowhood, old age or other lack of livelihood in circumstances beyond his control. (UN, 1948).

It could be argued then that human rights and disability rights are philosophically the same. However, there may often be instances in which disabled people are particularly affected by an issue which contravenes their rights. For instance, Andrew Lee, in the opening comments to this section, mentions being 'held back from engaging in life'.

Human rights are also about the right to life itself. For instance, in March 2006, human rights considerations were called into play by the High Court in London, in a case brought by the parents of a baby (known as Baby MB), who was being kept alive on a ventilator (BBC News, 2006). The child had a rare genetic condition, which would result in paralysis. His parents fought for his right to life, and in fact overruled the decision by medical personnel to turn off his ventilator. However, in a later case in 2009, another baby's right to life was similarly defended by his parents unsuccessfully (BBC News, 2009).

Human rights instruments can therefore have some effect on life-and-death decisions, but generic human rights statements cannot of themselves change society's institutions, nor can they ensure that discrimination does not happen. Indeed they are sometimes interpreted wrongly to mean that everyone should be treated in an identical way. An inquiry into access to health care by people with learning disabilities (Michael, 2008) identified poorer health outcomes for this group than for the rest of the population, and inattention to 'reasonable adjustments' of health services as a significant contributory factor. An example could be taken from GP (general practice) surgeries in the UK, which often assign appointment times of ten to fifteen minutes. Because people with learning disabilities might need much longer to understand and to express themselves, therefore they will effectively be denied their right to equal treatment through this uniform system. Over the past ten or twenty years, therefore, there has been a renewed interest in analysing how human rights can be put into action specifically for disabled people. In many cases, an adjustment or a specific process needs to be put into place, to ensure that human rights are upheld for all, and the word 'adjustment' therefore figured prominently in the UK Disability Discrimination Act 1995 (DDA 1995), discussed below.

A step forward for international human rights was made in 2007 with the UN Convention on the Rights of People with Disabilities, which has provided a fundamental shift in the way people with disabilities are viewed. It rejects the view of 'persons with disabilities as objects of charity, medical treatment and social protection' and affirms people with disabilities as:

> Subjects of rights, able to claim those rights as active members of society.
> (UN High Commissioner for Human Rights, 2008)

The Convention entered into force on 3 May 2008, and 109 very diverse countries have now ratified the convention, including the UK. The key principles are shown in Box 3.1.

Box 3.1	Principles of the UN Convention on the Rights of People with Disabilities (Article 3: UN, 2007)

a. Respect for inherent dignity, individual autonomy including the freedom to make one's own choices, and independence of persons;
b. Non-discrimination;
c. Full and effective participation and inclusion in society;
d. Respect for difference and acceptance of persons with disabilities as part of human diversity and humanity;
e. Equality of opportunity;
f. Accessibility;
g. Equality between men and women;
h. Respect for the evolving capacities of children with disabilities and respect for the right of children with disabilities to preserve their identities.

States ratifying the Convention are obliged to 'take all appropriate measures to eliminate discrimination on the basis of disability by any person, organization or private enterprise'. In the context of health and the right to life, we might note that this specifically includes measures to provide accessible information, and to promote staff training to ensure that these rights are put into practice. Further, governments are required to report to the international committee of the Convention on a regular basis, indicating progress in implementation. However it could still be maintained that some health services in the UK do in fact discriminate at an institutional level against people with learning disabilities. Human rights statements, in themselves, will not make a difference unless there is accompanying action to enforce them. Therefore, it is important to have mechanisms, guidance, laws and rules to put human rights into action.

Making human rights effective

One way of tackling human rights abuses is to outlaw practices which contravene human rights. Legislation about disability discrimination is a good example of this strategy, for instance the Americans with Disabilities Act (Department of Justice, 1990) which provided a framework of rights that were made concrete in anti-discrimination measures. In other words, if a person's right to an equal education was contravened, they could sue the education authority; if their right to access health services was not met, then they could take legal action. The British Disability Discrimination Act (1995) in some respects followed the American example, by defining what service providers and public bodies must do to adapt their services to disabled people. However, from the start, this Act was criticized by the UK disabled people's movement, since it appeared to lack 'teeth'. Those providing services were only required to make 'reasonable adjustments', and could themselves decide what that reasonableness consisted of. Despite being followed by specific disability duties, research in 2005 about the employment provisions of the Act (PIRU, 2005) found that it was very hard for disabled people to use the DDA 1995 in order to gain redress from public authorities, or employers.

Since then, thinking about equalities has shifted slightly in the UK, and the duty to make adjustments for disabled people is approached from the more generic standpoint of the disadvantages faced by a whole range of people, whose rights are regularly contravened in various ways. That includes people from different religions, races, people whose sexuality might single them out, as well as those who are disabled. The Equalities Unit in the UK government now overviews equality issues for all those groups, and in 2010 the Equality Act was passed, which replaces the DDA 1995. The three general duties of the Act are enforced by the 'specific duties' it puts on public bodies, to publish information to demonstrate their compliance, on an annual basis, and to set equality objectives at least every four years.

Box 3.2	General duties which public bodies must incorporate into their objectives under the Equality Act 2010 (Section 149)

(1) A public authority must, in the exercise of its functions, have due regard to the need to—

   (a) *eliminate discrimination*, harassment, victimisation and any other conduct that is prohibited by or under this Act;
   (b) *advance equality of opportunity* between persons who share a relevant protected characteristic and persons who do not share it;
   (c) *foster good relations* between persons who share a relevant protected characteristic and persons who do not share it.

[author's italic]

Much depends, of course, on the way in which this is put into action, and it is too early yet to say what effect it will have on the contravention of rights faced by people with learning disabilities. However, the Act specifically guides public authorities, including health services, that achieving equality for some groups of individuals may mean making special arrangements or adjustments to existing practices.

Human rights instruments, then, can provide a framework to approach all the topics in this book as they relate to the lives of people with learning disabilities. That is why a consideration of human rights should be at the forefront of practice in all spheres of life. This chapter will specifically examine the ways in which people with learning disabilities gain access to health services, before returning to some practice-related considerations about human rights, and how they can make a difference.

Research evidence about health care for people with learning disabilities

Health outcomes

Over the past thirty or forty years, views about health needs and learning disability have undergone a radical shift in the UK. Lesley Russ, a prominent health practitioner who has worked for many years with people with learning disabilities, looked back over the past decades to the time when she used to work as a community learning disability nurse:

> In the 1970s many people with learning disabilities lived in institutions, so health became the responsibility of those institutions, not of the families or of the individuals themselves. Those people's needs were often seriously neglected, and the climate of that time was that you didn't question doctors.[1]

Despite the shift in attitudes mentioned above, health outcomes for people with learning disabilities are still far from equitable in the Western world. Two systematic reviews of research (Alborz et al., 2005; Elliott et al., 2003) in the UK showed that many people with learning disabilities have basic unmet health needs and may access general practitioners (GPs) and dental surgeries less often than others. The particular factors identified were to do with physical access, communication problems between health professionals and patients, and provision shortage. The research reviewed by Elliott et al. (2003) particularly highlighted the significantly poorer health of people with learning disabilities than the general population in a number of priority areas such as mental health and dementia. Research had also revealed lower incidence of health checks for people with learning disabilities

---

[1] All quotations from Lesley Russ reproduced with her kind permission; conversation, 2009.

than for the general population, and poor collaboration between primary and secondary health services.

> Responding to the health inequalities faced by people with learning disabilities is a critically important issue for primary and secondary healthcare services in England. It is clear that these health inequalities are, to an extent, avoidable. (Emerson and Baines, 2010: 11)

The extent of health inequalities for people with learning disabilities in the UK was most dramatically illustrated by increased mortality rates in comparison to the general population (Tyrer et al., 2007). These authors analysed data for people with moderate to profound learning disability showing that both all-cause and disease specific mortality rates were over three times higher than those for the general population. Concurrently, Mencap drew attention to a series of case studies of people with profound learning disabilities who died in hospital; they highlighted serious failures in health care services for people with learning disabilities (Mencap, 2007), and argued that these deaths were all preventable. However, the causes of death were often complex and cannot simply be attributed to a non-responsive health service. Five years on, a follow-up report by Mencap (2012) detailed a further 74 cases of deaths which could have been preventable, and listed some of the possible system failures from families' points of view. Heslop et al. (2011) will report in 2013 on a full analysis of health pathways and factors which influenced the deaths of some 300 people with learning disabilities, thus giving us for the first time an evidence base and analytic insight into the systemic failures to meet their needs and also the possible ways to tackle these issues in the health care system.

Lifestyle, nutrition and exercise

People with learning disabilities are among the poorest in society in the UK today (Emerson et al., 2005). Based on quantitative evidence, Emerson and Hatton (2007b) conclude that socio-economic disadvantage may account for a high proportion of the health inequalities experienced by people with learning disabilities, both in terms of their physical and their mental health. As is the case with other socially excluded groups in the Western world, poverty can result in eating poor quality food, misuse of alcohol, and a lack of ability to maintain physical fitness (Taggart et al., 2006; McLaughlin et al., 2007).

Therefore, perhaps the greatest need for action is in the area of lifestyle issues; the choices we all make in our lives of course have an effect on our health, particularly in the areas of food and exercise. However, many people with learning disabilities have a poor diet and very low physical activity levels (Ells et al., 2006; Melville et al., 2007). They may, for instance, live in situations where it is not possible simply to get out and go for a walk; many people step straight from the home into a minibus. Compounded with this is the fact that food may be used as a source of pleasure and reward, or given as an easy route to a 'quiet life'. In-depth, interpretative research can help to understand that people with learning disabilities do not often exercise their own choice about such lifestyle issues, nor are they encouraged to learn and decide for themselves (Victoria Williams, 2011). Marshall *et al.* (2003) found 122 people had been identified for a weight reduction programme, but action had only been taken for 34 per cent of them. Melville *et al.* (2009) suggest that carers may have a low level of knowledge in these areas and also that their perceptions of the health benefits may differ from those of the people they support.

People with learning disabilities reflect some of the health issues common in the society in which they live. A serious issue in many Western countries is obesity, which is a significant factor leading to reduced life expectancy. Compared with the general population, obesity tends to occur at a younger age for people with learning disabilities, and will often lead to problems such as diabetes (Melville *et al.*, 2007). Moreover it should not be assumed that not being obese reflects a good nutritional diet as reviews of research in the UK (Ells *et al.*, 2006) conclude that fewer than one in ten people with learning disabilities have what could be called a 'healthy diet'. It should of course be remembered that the situation may be dramatically different in countries where many disabled people live in extreme poverty (Singal, 2010). In India, for example, where Singal's research took place, young disabled people struggled to have enough to eat. Lifestyle issues are tightly bound up with differences in culture and context. In some parts of the world, poverty and famine may be far more important issues than unhealthy eating.

Barriers in accessing health services

In the UK, the label 'learning disability', instead of ensuring specialist access to health care, unfortunately sometimes stands in the way of health care. This phenomenon is so common that it has a name, 'diagnostic overshadowing'. An example of what this means was given by Lesley Russ, based on her own experience in health promotion with people with learning disabilities:

> In one area I worked with a gentleman with a severe learning disability who went to see his GP, probably about 8 different times in less than 6 months. He lived with a brother who had a physical impairment, so getting to the surgery was not easy. Each time his brother reported different problems, such as skin rashes, bed wetting, itchy skin, weight loss and a leg ulcer. He visited his practice 8 times before someone tested his urine and found out he was diabetic. He was seen as a learning disabled man, not a man, a human being who needed to be looked at holistically. I don't believe there was wilful intent to neglect, but the learning disability was seen first. I believe it is called diagnostic overshadowing.

Clearly, this is a complex situation, and there are no easy answers. People with learning disabilities are often reliant on others to initiate their contact with health services, but even when this does happen there are many other obstacles which limit the quality of care provided for them in both primary and secondary care, including the following:

- Lack of physical access, transport to appointments and parking (Lennox *et al.*, 2003; Cumella and Martin, 2004).
- Lack of reliable and valid measures and assessments (Bollands and Jones, 2002; Ruddick and Oliver, 2005; Brown and MacArthur, 2006).
- Lack of knowledge of learning disability in mainstream health care professionals and appropriate staff training (Bollands and Jones, 2002; Wharton *et al.*, 2005; Brown and MacArthur, 2006).
- Communication problems between patient and clinicians (Ruddick, 2005; Wharton *et al.*, 2005).
- Poor collaboration between GPs, primary health care teams and specialist services (Bollands and Jones, 2002; Wharton *et al.*, 2005; Brown and MacArthur, 2006).
- Clinicians speaking to carers and not the patients (Lennox *et al.*, 2003).
- Lengthy appointment waiting times (Lennox *et al.*, 2003; Wharton *et al.*, 2005).

The central, and compounding, problems appear to be the difficulties some people may have in communicating their symptoms, and the lack of time and resources available to generic health providers, such as GPs or acute hospitals, in order to simply have enough time to listen, follow up concerns, and treat patients who may require extra support. These factors combine to make it extremely difficult for many people with learning disabilities to receive an equitable service from their doctor or their local hospital, and their own distress may then cause additional symptoms of anxiety.

Advances in medical treatments

Despite the emphasis so far on the ordinary health needs of people with learning disabilities, the situation is actually even more complex, with several interconnected factors affecting health. It is suggested by leading researchers that determinants of health inequalities can be divided into five main categories:

1. Increased risk of exposure to well established 'social determinants' of health.
2. Increased risk associated with specific genetic and biological causes of learning disabilities.
3. Communication difficulties and reduced health 'literacy'.
4. Personal health risks and behaviours.
5. Deficiencies in access to and the quality of healthcare provision.

(Emerson and Baines, 2010: 6)

Some of the factors in Emerson and Baines's list are to do with bio-medical factors associated with impairment. For instance, it is known that almost half of people with Down's syndrome have congenital heart defects (Brookes *et al.*,

1996), and the prevalence of epilepsy is at least twenty times higher among people with learning disabilities than in the general population (Kerr *et al.*, 2001).

Disability scholars have sometimes rejected medical 'cures' of disabling conditions, and indeed a learning disability in itself cannot readily be cured. However, Shakespeare (2006: ch. 7) argues for a more reasoned debate, which allows for the recognition of medical research and advances in specific areas, which can be of immense benefit to individuals who have particular conditions or syndromes. For instance, since the 1970s, the regular identification and dietary control of phenylketonuria (PKU), a genetic enzyme disease, has saved babies in the UK who could have been affected. This does not mean that people with PKU are devalued or denied the right to life, but simply that parents are given a choice to save their baby from immense problems in development and general health.

Bio-medical factors exist for individuals, alongside social and individual factors, and a moment's reflection will show how these factors can interact with each other. If it is known, for instance, that a particular population has a higher risk of developing hearing or visual impairments, then it is all the more necessary to ensure that: (a) the audiology clinics and optometrists are trained to meet their needs; (b) information is provided in such a way that people can understand. Similarly, people with learning disabilities who have a syndrome called Prader–Willi are prone to overeating, loss of muscle tone, and becoming overweight (Whittington and Holland, 2008). Medical advances have led to them enjoying longer lives, but their quality of life is vastly improved through correct social understanding of their condition and control of diet.

Complex health problems

Some people with learning disabilities do in fact have continuing and often complex health problems. For instance people with profound and multiple learning disabilities (see p. 18; Mansell, 2010) are prone to a range of specific health issues including:

- cerebral palsy resulting in low levels of movement control;
- sensory impairments; and
- difficulties in swallowing (dysphagia).

Carnaby (2004) also includes chronic pulmonary disease, and impairments in touch, pressure or detecting temperature and pain, which may complicate diagnosis and treatment. A combination of the above factors can result in a person being dependent on technology such as tube-feeding, and a complex array of supports for their very survival, as is outlined below:

> Some people may be described as having 'life limiting conditions'. Others have fragile health and can be susceptible to conditions like chest infections and gastro-intestinal problems. Good nutrition is vital for achieving good health, and skilled support is needed for feeding and swallowing in many cases. Many people experience a combination of

medical needs and need access to specialised health support to ensure they are holistically managed. (Dawkins, 2008)

There is an increasing number of infants born with such complex needs who are now able to survive into later childhood, adolescence or adulthood, due to advances in technological aids and intensive care regimes. In particular, the development of technology for tube feeding has enabled infants with very severe cerebral palsy and swallowing difficulties to have far healthier lives than before, as Townsley *et al.* (1999) explored. However, along with these technological advances come possible exclusions, since they can result in others feeling that they are not qualified to manage the technology. Parents and other family members may receive basic training, but they may find that their child is then held back from accessing educational or social venues, due to the need for 'trained medical staff' to be on hand. As people become older, other regulations about the health and safety of care staff may restrict individuals' lifestyle, such as bans on manual handling and lifting. Mencap has in fact run a campaign to lift such bans, so that people with profound and multiple learning difficulties (PMLD) are not denied the services that other people with learning disabilities can access. Nevertheless, this is a group who will need specific access to specialist health care, on a lifelong basis. That includes postural support and positioning, advice from physiotherapists, as well as technological support.

One family who had a baby – called Jack here, not his real name – with complex health care needs, was kind enough to provide information for this chapter. Their baby was born in 2006, and sadly died just before reaching the age of 2. However, they were determined to give their infant son the best life possible, and to enjoy him as an individual human being. Naturally, that meant involving many people, friends and family, but there were obstacles to overcome, as his mother, Anna, explained:

> He came (home from hospital) with a monitor that would alarm if the oxygen in his blood went down. So you'd run to his aid, so you didn't have to sit and watch him all the time, he was wired up. People were so scared of those things. We had to throw people in at the deep end, because it was really simple stuff. But we had to write lists and lists of procedures, but to me that was unnecessary. Once you knew how to suction and how to feed him, then the rest was nonsense. What was important was that you knew Jack. So that's why we kind of threw people in, so they could concentrate on him, rather than on those things that sounded really nasty.[2]

The trauma of supporting a child with complex needs was compounded for them by the way in which their baby was treated simply as a 'health care package', both by support staff and health professionals. For them, their infant was first and foremost a human being with a unique personality, and this is how they wanted him to

---

[2] Reproduced with kind permission of 'Anna'; personal conversation August 2009.

be treated by health professionals and others. There will be a whole array of health professionals involved with a baby with complex impairments, and this was indeed true for Jack and his family, who saw paediatricians, optometrists, hearing specialists, occupational and physiotherapists, gastric and respiratory specialists. While this level of service provision clearly represents the advances in medical science which have kept babies such as Jack alive, research about providing services for children and adults with complex health care needs has consistently echoed the need to coordinate services, to provide a key worker (Townsley *et al.*, 2004) and to engage with the person him or herself, rather than simply to see his health problems (Mansell, 2010). There is still a gap between health policy statements and practice.

Access to mental health support services

It is now well known that mental health distress is more likely to occur among people with learning disabilities than in the general population. This is particularly true among young people; the *Count Us In* enquiry (FPLD, 2002) found that 4 in 10 young people with learning disabilities will have a mental health support need at some point during adolescence. This statistic is supported by the literature generally, although the statistics do depend on the range of people who are 'counted in' (Hatton, 2002; Duggan and Brylewski, 1999).

The action research projects which followed the *Count Us In* enquiry found that mental health and learning disability services were not well 'joined up'. This meant in practice that people who had the label of learning disability were not readily recognized as needing mental health support. Williams and Heslop (2005, 2006) found that a mental health need was often diagnosed only when the problem became obvious through behavioural challenges or anger.

While access to mental health services therefore remains a problem for many people with learning disabilities, their problems are more readily attributed to 'challenging behaviour', and psychotropic medication is then administered which is both poorly understood and often inappropriate (Heslop, 2006). The possibility of emotional distress is often ignored, as people with learning disabilities have traditionally been considered to lack emotional depth (Arthur, 2003). However, in a subsequent interview-based study, Heslop and Macaulay (2009) examined the views of people with learning disabilities who self-injured. The twenty-five people who took part in the research were able to express the depth of the difficulties they had experienced, although sometimes these issues had not been taken seriously by those around them. Interestingly, their preferred ways of being supported were no different to those preferred by people without a learning disability:

> Most participants particularly valued having someone to talk with, and/or someone to listen to them. They also expressed another three key features of helpful support regarding their self-injury. These were:

> ■ the provision of sensitive support in looking after their injuries, such as practical help with cleaning their wounds and accessing dressing materials;
> ■ help to change their ways of thinking, not their ways of behaving; and

■ knowing that they were not alone and/or having contact with someone else who self-injured. (Heslop and Macaulay, 2009: 3)

Human rights in practice: improving access to health care

Quite simply, we cannot hope to improve people's health and well-being if we are not ensuring their human rights are respected. (Rosie Winterton MP, 2007, Joint Committee on Human Rights: Eighteenth Report)

Taking control of your own health

If health care and equality of health outcomes are human rights issues, then the research evidence above shows that, for a variety of reasons, people with learning disabilities in general often fail to have their rights met. However, this is clearly a complex picture, in which biological predisposition, personal responsibility, as well as access to health services all play a role. It is worth reiterating that a human rights perspective is not just about delivering everything in the same way to everyone; if that happened with health services, people with learning disabilities would often miss out. For instance, a man with complex behavioural challenges will need consideration, time and good support to go into hospital for an operation. For different reasons, people with learning disabilities living in the community may miss out on public health campaigns, such as the 'Change 4 Life' campaign (NHS, 2012), which aims to combat obesity by delivering recipe cards to people's homes. For some people, these may be difficult to read, and for others, they may assume access to ingredients, resources and expertise that are not available to those who are living in poverty.

One central way of considering how to redress the human rights issues about health is to consider how people could be more in control of their own lives, and how at least some could take greater responsibility for their own health, or could work collectively to increase the accountability of health services. For instance, in many areas in England and Wales, there are now teams of people with learning disabilities set up as 'health trainers', whose role is to monitor health services locally and also to take a part in educating medical practitioners. A 'good practice' example highlighted in the revised guidance to Health Action Planning issued by the Department of Health in 2009 (DH, 2009b) pulls together strategic thinking and the involvement of people with learning disabilities themselves:

Box 3.3	Good practice example from Guidance to Health Action Planning (2009)

Bath and North East Somerset PCT have appointed a learning disability nurse (who has an MA in public health) within their public health department. She works closely with self-advocates to make sure people with learning disabilities benefit from local and national public health initiatives. Recent work includes local activities to increase awareness of the use and dangers of salt in food.

Source: DH, 2009b: 32

At an individual level, one of the most important ways of tackling the multiple health problems facing people with learning disabilities in the UK is the idea of health action planning (often known as HAPs), which was introduced formally in 2002, following the 2001 Learning Disability strategy, *Valuing People*. A health action plan is defined as:

> The actions needed to maintain and improve the health of an individual and any help needed to accomplish these. It is a mechanism to link the individual and the range of services and supports they need if they are to have better health ... the plan is primarily for the person with learning disabilities and is usually co-produced with them. (DH, 2009a: 4)

How does a health action plan work? In many ways, the idea of health action planning is about a process, rather than an actual product. Although many areas have introduced accessible 'templates' or health books to support people's planning, it is quite possible to carry out a plan for health in many different ways, resulting in (for instance):

- a photo booklet about health choices;
- a video to remind you about the decisions you have made relating to eating or lifestyle;
- a booklet to show health professionals what types of health needs you have; and
- a collection of reminders for people to be able to communicate their health needs to professionals.

Health passports are another form of health action planning, in which patients can note down key information that is essential for others to know, particularly in an emergency.

Providing specific health checks for people with learning disabilities

Health action plans are clearly insufficient on their own. A patient with learning disabilities cannot be 'in control' of his or her own health, if the doctor does not listen or if their appointment is not long enough. Alongside health action planning, therefore, systemic solutions also need to be sought, which seek to address directly the barriers that have been identified in the ways in which health services are delivered.

The provision of annual health checks set up for people with learning disabilities specifically appears to be beneficial (Martin, 2003; Baxter *et al.*, 2006). All these studies demonstrated positive effects, including the fact that these checks highlighted treatable conditions that may not have received attention. Cassidy *et al.* (2002) found that 94 per cent of people with learning disabilities attending their first check had a physical health problem warranting intervention, and Robertson *et al.* (2010) summarize the evidence for the effectiveness of GP led health checks for all people with learning disabilities. Houghton has developed a step-by-step guide for GP practices. Enabling people with learning disabilities to have equal and effective access to health care is a partnership process, as Houghton explains:

> The combination of providing a multidisciplinary health care assessment (with practice nurse and doctor involved) will maximise the quality and the health outcomes for the person with learning disabilities. (2010: 21)

Health checks therefore appear to constitute an effective intervention requiring minimal staff time, training and additional costs, although a systematic review of evidence reported that, while the number of health checks has increased, the average uptake in England is still only about 50 per cent and there are wide variations between areas (Robertson *et al.*, 2010).

Altering existing arrangements to suit people with learning disabilities

If access to primary health care is fraught with problems for people with learning disabilities, they may face equal barriers in a hospital admission, or indeed in seeing a specialist in relation to community dental, audiology or eye specialists. This barrier particularly applies to those with the highest level of additional health problems, namely those with complex or profound needs. The problems identified in hospital admissions include anxiety about the stay, exacerbated by lack of information and emotional support (Bollands and Jones, 2002; Cumella and Martin, 2004). There are inadequate facilities for those with complex needs, and it seems that often the only way in which some people with learning disabilities can access ordinary hospital care is for their family members or carers to provide constant practical support (Wharton *et al.*, 2005).

A human rights approach would lead to plans for 'reasonable adjustments', so that these problems can be overcome, and sometimes quite simple measures can improve matters. For instance, one study (Hannon, 2004) explored hospital pre-admission assessments for people with learning disabilities by community liaison nurses. All the participants' experiences of their admission were better than expected. The participants described being treated the same as other patients and being satisfied with the standards of cleanliness and food. Carers reported good support from the hospital staff, who in their turn were very positive about the input from the community nurses. There were some negative issues such as doctors not speaking directly to the patients, but overall it appeared that the pre-admission liaison work was effective in making the hospital stay a more positive experience.

Similarly, the uptake of services such as eye examinations and dental checks is much lower for people with learning disabilities than for the general population. However, when Starling *et al.* (2006) offered eye tests to a cohort of adults with learning disabilities they found it was possible to undertake this with all those who accepted. Some people with profound learning disabilities needed to be assessed at home and some could not use conventional tests, but an adequate examination was successful for everybody.

An important advance in many general hospitals in England is the introduction of a hospital liaison nurse (Garvey, 2008), who may have specific responsibility for advising other health care staff about the needs of patients with a learning disability (Kerr *et al.*, 2009. As Garvey (2008) describes, 'the role focuses not only on working directly with clinicians and patients, supporting care delivery and providing advice, but also on raising the profile of the support available to adults through community teams and specialist services for this group'. A specialist nurse often has a specific role in ensuring medical practitioners understand the communication of a particular patient, and they can also be key to making links with professionals outside the health care setting, ensuring smoother discharge arrangements.

Providing accessible information

One of the most widespread barriers to inclusion, which faces nearly all people with learning disabilities, is the dominance of written information in everyday life. Even for those who can read, complex and abstract expressions will tend to make things difficult for most people with learning disabilities. Therefore, the 'translation' of information into accessible formats is often considered to be an important factor in working to redress human rights issues. Like all the other themes in this book, it should not just be left to specialists: all the partners involved in helping someone with their health can become more effective by learning the basics about accessible information.

The DDA 1995, now replaced by the Equality Act 2010 makes it unlawful to discriminate against a disabled person in respect to goods and services, which include provision of information. Access to information is a human right, and therefore where there are difficulties in understanding or reading, then information providers are required by law to provide that information in suitable formats. However, practice is more difficult than theory. Everyone is different, and what is accessible to one person may not meet another person's needs, as emphasized in the guidance produced by the project *Information for All* (Rodgers *et al.*, 2004).

Whether providing information for just one person, or for a whole population, the first task has to be to work out what information is actually needed (Rodgers *et al.*, 2004). Some points may be irrelevant, and others may be confusing for the reader. Therefore, most accessible forms of information are in fact summaries of the 'main points'. Second, the translator has to work with the text. This involves making it clear what exactly the words are supposed to mean. It often means converting a long, embedded sentence into straightforward, active sentences with a subject and a verb. For instance, the sentence: 'For low-cost recipes, healthy eating tips, super deals and more, you'll find everything you need to refresh your

Figure 3.1	Individual needs for information (fictional examples from different projects)
Jane could decode written text well, and read out loud in a meaningful way. However, at the end of her reading, she often did not know what she had read. At the end of another day, she would have forgotten the information entirely.	Jane needs someone to double-check with her, and to explain things in a different way to check her understanding. She may also need a system for recalling the points to remember, such as a notebook or pile of cards with a few words on each one.
Marcus could make out most simple words, but had difficulty with longer words or those which were unfamiliar. He would get lost when faced with dense text.	It would be best to simplify the text for Marcus, and pick out the key points he really needs. The text could also be presented in chunks, with a picture by each chunk.
Maria could not read much at all. However, she understood and communicated well verbally.	Maria might prefer to have her information in an audio format, such as a CD or an audio file.
Jake had very low levels of attention, and was extremely active and energetic. When presented with pictures, he tended to tear them up; however, he did relate to written language and loved computers.	It would be useful for Jake to have information on the computer, and perhaps to find websites which would mean something to him. Some accessible websites have auditory components, which might also help Jake.

menu here' (NHS, 2012) could be translated as: 'Look at this website. You will find recipes for cheap meals. You can find out about healthy eating.' Pictures, symbols or photos are also regularly used, and there is an array of resources for making easy information at the end of this chapter, and in particular, readers may find the website 'Easy Health' (easyhealth.org.uk) very useful.

Changing attitudes

The barriers to receiving equal health treatment are not simply about physical access, nor even about information. They are also about attitudes of medical professionals, and nowhere is this better illustrated than by a consideration of mental health issues. Like many other health issues considered in this chapter, mental health distress has to be taken seriously when people with learning disabilities experience it, in order for them to be 'included' within health services. Their access to a healthy life requires a shift in thinking, so that problems are *not* just attributed to the learning disability. Instead, professionals and support staff need to recognize that people with learning disabilities are no different from others in the community in needing ready access to health services.

An emotionally healthy lifestyle for people with learning disabilities has two aspects:

1. Prevention of emotional distress through tackling the root problems, such as lack of friends and isolation (Arthur 2003; Williams and Heslop, 2005).
2. Access to responsive and helpful mental health services for those who need them.

Research carried out at Norah Fry Research Centre (Williams and Heslop, 2006; Heslop, 2006; Heslop and Macaulay, 2009) has focused on ways in which mental health distress is seen not just as 'pathology', but more as a reaction to the difficulties people face in their lives. The human rights agenda, for instance, leads to questions about whether people are having their rights met in accessing health care, but also whether they are treated with 'respect for inherent dignity, individual autonomy including the freedom to make one's own choices', or indeed whether they are granted 'full and effective participation and inclusion in society' (Principles 1 and 3 of the UN Convention; UN, 2007). This does not imply, of course, that mental health support is unnecessary, but the human rights agenda may lead to less invasive, more person-centred ways of approaching support than psychotropic medication. It may also lead practitioners to ensure that people's lives are viewed in holistic ways, in which they have the maximum control and choice in all aspects.

Conclusion: what have human rights achieved for health services?

This chapter started with consideration of 'the right to life', and this strikes at the heart of how learning disability is seen in society at large. Are the lives of people with learning disabilities given equal value with those of others in society, and how is this value reflected in the health care they receive and indeed their health outcomes? The evidence summarized in this chapter unfortunately implies that the human rights of people with learning disabilities are still routinely denied in the UK, in this fundamental area of their lives. The application of human rights considerations to health care is of course a sensitive matter, since with increasingly expensive and sophisticated treatments, rationing may have to occur. There is no automatic right to choose whether or not to have a particular treatment, despite the current emphasis on patient choice. Further, no one can have a right to 'be healthy', even if there is a human right to adequate medical care, as discussed above. Nevertheless, a violation of human rights does occur if people's lives are devalued, if they automatically go to the back of the queue, or if a medical condition is not recognized or treated in the same way as it would for anyone else in society. The evidence of increased mortality in people with learning disabilities, and premature, preventable deaths, indicates that the human rights agenda is still very important as a standard by which to judge our health services.

Human rights statements on their own however will not ensure that people with learning disabilities receive better health care. It is the legal obligation to make 'reasonable adjustments' to services that will improve access, and that is why it is important to understand exactly what adjustments are required in health care for people with learning disabilities. The evidence points to certain adjustments which have proved successful, such as liaison nurses in general hospitals, and annual health checks for people with learning disabilities. All these need to be implemented in a more systematic way, and further knowledge will help to understand exactly what the barriers and solutions may be. The Department of Health is funding a three-year public health observatory (2010–13) to investigate what exactly does lead to poor health outcomes for people with learning disabilities. As mentioned above, research at the Norah Fry Research Centre in Bristol (Heslop *et al.*) will report in 2013 on findings from a confidential inquiry into the care pathways of people with learning disabilities who have died in one geographical area of England over a two-year period. Some of the adjustments required will require shifts in practice, others will require a rethink in attitudes, and many will require reskilling medical practitioners about how to communicate with patients who may have particular communication needs.

As the basis for policy, the notion of human rights is sometimes misunderstood and critiqued; individual cases of human rights violations can seem to imply an impossible task for an already overstretched health service. Yet some of the adjustments and solutions highlighted in this chapter are not expensive to implement. Improved information and communication for instance are simply about the professional skills of practitioners, and about giving slightly more time and consideration to particular patients. Adopting a human rights perspective does *not* mean treating everyone in exactly the same way. It is about the recognition and valuing of differences, and the delivery of health services so that each person with learning disabilities can enjoy a life that is maximally healthy.

Reflection exercises

1. A useful way to address some of the issues and tensions discussed in this chapter would be to think about a particular person with learning disabilities, and to track through with them their encounters with health services and their attitudes to health. Some people with learning disabilities may have had frequent hospitalization and visits to the doctor, while others will have remained relatively healthy. However, they are all likely to have encountered some barriers in accessing health services.

2. A person with learning disabilities recently said that she wanted to move to a downstairs flat, since there had been a fire, and she was unable to use the lift. She was advised to go and talk to her psychologist. Think about why this type of anomaly happens, and what lies beneath it.

3. It is often hard for people with learning disabilities to know what symptoms matter, and when/how they should contact a medical practitioner. If you are a practitioner, consider how you can work with others to ensure that a person's symptoms are reported promptly.

4. Human rights and lifestyle choices pose some challenges. Review what these may be, by considering the eating and exercise habits that you yourself and your friends may adopt, and compare these with a person with learning disabilities you know.

Suggested further resources

1. To follow up information concerning human rights, a good place to start is the British Institute of Human Rights (BIHR) (2006) *Your Human Rights: A Guide for Disabled People*, at: bigwww.bihr.org.uk/resources/guides

2. For those who are making easy information about health matters, the guides to accessible information can be found at:

   www.bristol.ac.uk/norahfry/research/completed-projects/infoforall.pdf

   These do not provide a 'how to do it' set of instructions, but they do offer a set of principles to guide those who are preparing information for people with learning disabilities in any language.

3. www.easyhealth.org.uk gives a very useful index of symbols and pictures that can be used in health information.

4. www.apictureofhealth.southwest.nhs.uk has a range of resources and easy information to help practitioners and has specific sections on different areas such as mental health and acute hospitals.

5. For access to the latest information about health for people with learning disabilities, the Health Observatory materials and publications can be found at:

   www.improvinghealthandlives.org.uk

6. A step-by-step guide to annual health checks for people with learning disabilities can be found at: www.rcgp.org.uk

4 Inclusion in Education

Inclusion is a key theme in government policy in the UK, where it is often seen as the converse of 'social exclusion'. Chapter 4 is about inclusion and young people with learning difficulties. It aims to explore what inclusion means specifically within the context of education.

Key points summary:

- It is a human right to be included in education. We can tell what the wider society is like by looking at its schools and colleges.
- All children are different and have individual needs. They should all have a place and be valued for who they are.
- Schools and colleges are told they have to include students with learning difficulties. But schools also have to get better exam results. It is sometimes hard for schools to do both.
- Children should all have a voice about their own learning and their lives.
- Inclusion can mean different things. It may be about learning together in one school, but it can also mean that everyone has a good education that meets their own needs.

Introduction and overview

 Voice of Experience

Everyone is different really which I think is good.
Otherwise it would be boring.
You must be allowed to be who you are.
I am never alone, never feel that way,
even though the others seem to think so.
They don't really know what I feel.

Source: disabled child in inclusive classroom, in Nilholm and Alm, 2010: 248

Inclusion in the mainstream of education, it is argued here, is a universal right. For example the recent UN Convention on the Rights for Persons with Disabilities emphasizes that:

> (states should) ensure an inclusive education system at all levels and life long learning directed to:
>
> (a) The full development of human potential and sense of dignity and self-worth, and the strengthening of respect for human rights, fundamental freedoms and human diversity;
> (b) The development by persons with disabilities of their personality, talents and creativity, as well as their mental and physical abilities, to their fullest potential;
> (c) Enabling persons with disabilities to participate effectively in a free society. (UN, 2007: Article 24)

One of the fundamental human rights, as seen, is the right to be included in society and within one's own community. This chapter now focuses on how that concept of 'inclusion' can be shaped, particularly in the context of childhood and education. Inclusion is a problematic and shifting concept, as we shall explore in the next section of this chapter.

Julian Goodwin, in the opening story in Chapter 1, recalled how pleased he was to be placed in a mainstream high school in America. Although he had previously made the most of his stay in a UK residential special school, his main point was that 'I didn't learn much that was useful to me'. Access to a more challenging, and useful, curriculum should also therefore be part of inclusive education. Inclusion for children with learning difficulties is far from universal, and has certainly not long been the norm in the UK. Until 1970 children who would now be labelled as having 'severe learning difficulties' were considered ineducable, and were not part of the education system at all. Instead, their school days were spent either in hospital schools or in 'junior training centres', which were the childhood version of 'adult training centres' or day centres for adults with learning disabilities. The right to universal education is thus culturally determined, and the Western notion of 'inclusion' might still work out very differently in other countries (Urwick and Elliott, 2010; Miles and Singal, 2010). Even in the UK, the idea of inclusion shifts according to prevailing attitudes:

> What we resolve to do in school only makes sense when considered in the broader context of what the society intends to accomplish through its educational investment in the young. How one conceives of education, we have finally come to recognize, is a function of how one conceives of culture and its aims, professed and otherwise. (Bruner, 1996: ix–x)

Although definitions of 'learning disability' have already been discussed in Chapter 2, it is necessary to revisit these briefly in this chapter. The first point to note is that the preferred term in an educational context is 'learning difficulty', and so that is the terminology used in this chapter. As mentioned in Chapter 2 (pp. 14–15), intelligence testing is generally regarded by educational psychology as only one, very limited tool, in a dynamic assessment process. In other words, the assessment of 'learning difficulty' is made within the context of a particular school system, and focuses largely on what can be done to foster learning (Frederickson and Cline, 2002: 252–8). The education system nevertheless plays a key role in defining who counts as having a 'learning difficulty', and also uses the term in a slightly different way than in adult services, leading to the language of special education needs becoming 'highly contentious and confusing', as noted by Ofsted (2010: 8–9). Confusions are a result of the following factors:

1. 'Special educational needs' (SEN), as defined in the 1981 Education Act, does not just refer to learners with learning difficulties. It is a wider category, which comprises children who may have a need for extra support due to a variety of factors, including emotional and behavioural difficulties, dyslexia and other specific learning difficulties.
2. It is usually at school age that the assessment process will take place, by virtue of which a child's status as having a 'learning difficulty' is first introduced. While the assessment is geared towards matching appropriate educational provision to the child's needs, it also has the much wider effect of giving the child a particular social status of difference in their family and social life outside the school.
3. The number of individuals defined as having a 'learning difficulty' at school age is larger than those who will receive adult services by virtue of having a learning *disability*. The demands of an education system create a category of people who find academic skills difficult, but may manage other aspects of their lives with a degree of independence.
4. Finally, the category of learning difficulty, and/or special educational need, is often falsely inflated by the over-representation of children who find learning difficult because their home language and culture are different, or indeed are recent immigrants or refugees.

(Dyson and Gallannaugh, 2008)

All these factors together result in a far larger population of children with SEN (see Box 4.1 for a definition), as compared with adults who have learning disabilities. This chapter often concerns itself with the whole SEN group, since in practice there is often no need to differentiate within that group. When certain points refer to particular sub-groups, that will be made explicit.

The next section of this chapter discusses 'inclusion' as a framework for reflection and practice, and considers what the word might mean. The chapter then moves on to give an overview of educational inclusion for children with SEN, from the point of view of research evidence.

In common with Barton (2003) and Lindsay (2003), this chapter considers inclusive education as a human right. Therefore, research to measure the extent to which inclusive policies work is, to a large extent, irrelevant. However, there has been a significant research focus on understanding more precisely the basis of

> **Box 4.1** **Definition of Special Educational Needs**
>
> Children have special educational needs if they have a *learning difficulty* which calls for *special educational provision* to be made for them. Children have a *learning difficulty* if they:
>
> (a) have a significantly greater difficulty in learning than the majority of children of the same age; or
> (b) have a disability which prevents or hinders them from making use of educational facilities of a kind generally provided for children of the same age in schools within the area of the local education authority
> (c) are under compulsory school age and fall within the definition at (a) or (b) above or would so do if special educational provision was not made for them.
>
> *Source*: Revised Code of Practice, DCSF 2001a

intervention in the early years of childhood, what hinders educational inclusion in later years, and what children's own experiences of education can tell us. The final part of the chapter will then consider some of the evidence about what works: how can the notion of inclusive education really make a difference to children with learning difficulties?

Key policy concept: inclusion

Inclusion and a social model of childhood disability

Inclusion as a concept is closely allied with the ideas of social model theorists, such as Oliver (1990) as discussed in Chapter 2. Throughout, this book adopts an essentially 'social model' view, of the relationship between individuals, impairments and environments. In this view, although children with SEN may have inherent problems with certain aspects of learning, nevertheless, educators need to ensure that they do not simply consider that the child with SEN constitutes a 'problem' that has to be fitted into an existing structure. Instead, a social model view puts the emphasis on systemic changes in the school, which should shift and reform to encompass the needs of *all* its pupils.

Disabled children have not always been accounted for, as part of the social model (Stalker and Connors, 2007). Not only are they devalued as being children and irresponsible to speak for their own rights, but they have had the double disadvantage of being disabled, and seen as a burden on resources. Shakespeare and Watson (1998) therefore propose a social model of childhood disability, in which the barriers faced by disabled children are seen as the segregation and oppression they receive from society generally. Yet it is hard to account for all the problems faced by a child with learning difficulties, without having some recourse to ideas about their own deficits and inherent differences. A 'relational' or interactional view (Norwich, 2002; Wendelborg and Tossebro, 2010) bridges the divide between social and medical, and acknowledges the importance of defining the exact relationship between individual needs and strengths, and the whole system or environment of the school in which the child takes part.

> Learning problems are a result of the relationship between issues that are specific to the individual and the demands, pressures and support that derive from the wider environment. (Wendelborg and Tossebro, 2010: 703)

The school environment for instance could exacerbate the problems faced by a child with learning difficulties, since they may find it harder than other children to adapt to rules of behaviour in a large group. However, a teacher could take pains to explain and remind children (for example, using visual rules) of how to behave in the classroom, and the child with learning difficulties may thereby benefit by knowing how and why to seek help (see the Teachers' TV example in resources section at end of this chapter).

What is inclusion in education?

Inclusion of children with learning difficulties is often, wrongly, taken to mean that a disabled child is placed within an ordinary school, perhaps with extra support, but without any major systemic changes within the school. However, inclusive education is more than simply 'putting disabled children into mainstream schools'. Education both mirrors and feeds into society, and as such it has to be seen as a political force (Slee, 2010; Barton, 2003). Many proponents of inclusion take this wider, political view, and would argue that inclusion must imply valuing the differences offered by all children, not simply giving special support to the children who are labelled as having a 'learning difficulty'.

> Inclusive education is part of a human rights approach to social relations and conditions. The intentions and values involved relate to a vision of the whole society of which education is a part. (Barton, 2003: 59)

If some children are segregated in special schools, that too is a political act, as it reflects the segregationist attitude of a wider society that does not value or include them. Education can both contribute to the disablement of young people, but conversely it can also contribute to their liberation and to the reshaping of a society in which all young people have a valued place.

Box 4.2 illustrates this wider, political view of inclusion in education, as proposed by the Alliance for Inclusive Education. According to this clear vision, inclusion in education is about broad inclusion in society, and about a society that values differences and diversity. It follows that inclusion in school both draws on wider societal discourses and helps to shape those discourses.

Box 4.2	**The Alliance for Inclusive Education defines nine principles of inclusion in education:**

- A person's worth is independent of their abilities or achievements
- Every human being is able to feel and think
- Every human being has a right to communicate and be heard
- All human beings need each other
- Real education can only happen in the context of real relationships
- All people need support and friendship from people of their own age
- Progress for all learners is achieved by building on things people can do rather than what they can't
- Diversity brings strength to all living systems
- Collaboration is more important than competition

Source: Alliance for Inclusive Education, 2010

The policy and legal basis for inclusion in education in the UK

As mentioned above, the right to education for disabled children in England started in 1970, with the inclusion of all children in the education system itself. However, the moves towards 'mainstream' inclusion started in earnest with a raft of research leading to the report by Warnock (1978), which proposed a new vision for British schools. The concept of special educational needs (SEN) stems from Warnock, who suggested that about one in five children would have SEN at some point in their school career, a far greater proportion of the school population than had previously been recognized as in need of support. The 1981 Education Act thus allowed schools to provide particular supports to a vast number of children, who were now defined as having 'SEN', and who could be educated, theoretically, in the mainstream. It also introduced the idea of a 'statement of special educational needs', which set out the support and adjustments required by a child with SEN, in some respects giving families the right to insist on schools providing what was indicated on the statement. However, the progress towards actual mainstream placements was slow. Some twenty-five years later, more than a third of children with statements of SEN were still educated in special schools:

- 242,500 (or 2.9 per cent of) pupils across all schools in England had statements of SEN, although around 18% of all pupils were categorised as having some type of special educational need.
- Of those with statements, 60% were in maintained mainstream schools (nursery, primary, secondary)
- 37.2% were in state-run special schools
- The remaining pupils with statements of SEN were mostly in pupil referral units (PRUs).

(House of Commons Education and Skills Committee, 2006: 28)

Since the early 1990s, repeated policies have broadly promoted inclusion in schools across the UK, and more recently in England and Wales. In England, the 1993 Education Act gave local education authorities (LEAs) the duty to place children in mainstream schools: (a) if it was appropriate to the child's needs; (b) did not conflict with the interests of other children; and (c) was an efficient use of the LEA's resources. Schools had to have SEN policies and explain how they would ensure equal treatment of disabled children. In 1994, this was followed by a Code of Practice, revised in 1996 and again in 2001.

The Code of Practice urged schools themselves to take as much responsibility as possible for all children, including those with SEN, and introduced the role of 'special educational needs coordinator' (SENCO) in each secondary school. The Code also emphasized the rights of all children to access the national curriculum, and promoted the idea of partnership between parents, schools, LEAs and other services. At international level, the UNESCO Salamanca Statement (1994) emphasized the idea that local mainstream schools should be open to *all pupils*, 'unless there are compelling reasons for doing otherwise'.

Legislation about inclusion has also played a role, since the 1993 Education Act, and significantly the 2001 Special Educational Needs and Disability Act, which built on the Disability Discrimination Act 1995, by making it illegal for education providers to discriminate against disabled pupils. The 2001 Act required schools and local authorities to plan strategically, to increase access for all pupils with SEN. Schools had to make appropriate arrangements for admission, not refuse an application on the grounds of disability, nor exclude pupils for reasons relating to their disability.

Since 2001, educational policy about including children with SEN has been more generic, recognizing that there are wider issues for all children who may be vulnerable or at risk. In 2003, *Every Child Matters* reflected the growing concerns about children who were abused, or needed protection by the state, and established the five fundamental outcomes for all children, which are:

1. Be healthy
2. Stay safe
3. Enjoy and achieve
4. Make a positive contribution
5. Achieve economic well-being

However, the campaign Every Disabled Child Matters pointed out in 2006 the continued discrepancy between the outcomes planned for *all* children, and those obtained by disabled children and their families. One answer to this problem is to envisage the school as one part only of a wider range of services and supports, which effectively create a 'team around the child', as put forward in the Children's Plan 2007. Whether they are mainstream or special, this vision puts schools in a central position, communicating with other partners, and taking a more holistic view of the child. The 2009 report of the Lamb Inquiry (DCSF, 2009) took further the notion of partnership, by a renewed emphasis on working with parents and families, and indeed empowering them to choose for their child. In some respects, of course, this idea of choice can undermine the move towards inclusion, since some parents may choose to have their children educated in special schools. Indeed, the 2011 Green Paper (DCSF, 2011) confirms that change in the tide, by proposing the location of education matters less than ensuring that each child has their educational needs met appropriately:

> There should be real choice for parents and that is why we are committed to removing any bias towards inclusion that obstructs parent choice and preventing the unnecessary closure of special schools. (2.46)

Despite this large volume of policy reports, inquiries and consultations, the achievement of inclusion has not been totally resolved, and indeed the very definition is still both contentious and difficult to grasp. The notion of 'inclusion' can take on a narrow meaning and indeed can be blamed for the lack of appropriate schooling for some children. This swings the pendulum back to the importance of ensuring a wide range of choices of educational provision, with an emphasis instead on the rights to inclusion in the fundamental outcomes for all children. The question remains each time a child with learning difficulties reaches school age: can an education system be developed in which all children are valued, their differences recognized, and their individual needs met?

An inclusive system or inclusive classrooms?

The vision of an inclusive society is not necessarily reflected in popular uses of the term 'inclusion' where it usually refers only to children with SEN/disabilities being accepted and included in ordinary classrooms. This definition is now seen to be both simplistic and problematic for several reasons. Positioning inclusive schooling as the opposite to segregated schooling conceals many traps. If children with SEN are simply placed in ordinary classrooms without appropriate attention to their support, then the result can often be that their differences are emphasized. Critics of inclusion will then state that those children are placing unnecessary and intolerable demands on the system, and that their education in any case would be better served in separate provision. However, the UK government definition of inclusion is consistent with an idea of an 'inclusive system', rather than 'inclusive, ordinary classrooms':

> Inclusion is about the quality of a child's experience and providing access to the high quality education which enables them to progress with their learning and participate fully in the activities of their school and community. (DfES, 2006: section 28)

An inclusive system of education is, first and foremost, one in which every child has a right to receive an education suited to their own needs. According to those arguments, it is possible for a child with learning difficulties to be 'included in education', while having their own educational programme within an environment that suits them. However, the political implications of inclusion have to be borne in mind. As an educational psychologist in Bristol, UK commented:

'Inclusion also seems generally to be cast in the role of having to justify itself, so that if it's not "perfect", then special school must be better ... but to me, what needs justifying is why you should separate and segregate.'[1]

It is important to recall the lessons learned about apartheid, where black people were kept out of public places, such as libraries or leisure centres – and, of course, schools. It may be that there are parallels here with inclusion for disabled children, if inclusion is seen in the context of power. The act of being shut out from society's mainstream institutions is an act of oppression, since it is something done by the powerful to the powerless. This chapter will concern itself with arguments about how that situation can be changed, but before that, the following section will examine some of the trends in research evidence about inclusion in the early years, and on entry into the school system.

Research about inclusive education

Early intervention and 'compensatory' programmes

Including children with learning difficulties in the education system is often a matter of considering both social and biological factors in tandem. For instance, recent advances in neuroscience (Della Sala and Anderson, 2012) have allowed educators to understand more precisely the identification and timing of some of the barriers to learning faced by young children with learning difficulties. Although these authors stress the pitfalls in uncritically translating neuroscience into education, the volume illustrates how psychology, education and neuroscience can be brought together. For instance, it is now understood that there are sensitive periods of brain development, during which it is crucial to have the input needed for development. There is evidence of remarkable synaptic growth during the first three months of life, and thereafter the following two years constitute a sensitive period both for language and perceptual development, when it is especially important for adult input to match or slightly outstrip the child's, staying within his or her 'zone of proximal development' (Vygotsky, 1987).

Taken together, these theories underline how important it is to get educational provision right from an early age. They also point out some possible additional problems for those whose development does not follow the norm. Where a child's language development, for instance, lags several years behind that of their peers, then adults may find it harder to adapt their input to the child's individual level. This may also apply to infants who are not developing normally, since the period at which they need the close 'parent–baby' contact, which comes naturally in infancy, may not occur until much later in life (Geekie and Raban, 1994).

Early intervention programmes thus seek to support and develop the environment surrounding young children who have learning difficulties, both in the

---

[1] All quotations from Carmel Hand, Educational Psychologist, reproduced with her kind permission; personal conversation, November 2008.

home (e.g. Portage service: Russell, 2011) and in pre-school programmes such as 'Sure Start'. Springate *et al.* (2008) reviewed the evidence on outcomes for all vulnerable groups of children, following early years interventions, and found evidence of improvements in cognitive development and social/behavioural outcomes, as well as health outcomes in the short term, with some evidence that these would be sustained in adult life. The crucial factor here is family input, and so services are often set up to support the family, so that they can become experts in finding ways to help their own child (Townsley *et al.*, 2004). This type of service does not imply that parents are at fault, or inadequate, in supporting their own children. On the contrary, support services for families should be about sharing expertise with parents and treating them as equals in the effort to find solutions for their child (see Chapter 5).

While there is some consensus, then, that early intervention matters, it is also important to consider the effect of these intervention programmes on the inclusion of children with learning difficulties in ordinary pre-school provision. At this early stage, it is not simply 'special input' that is necessary, but a context in which the child can develop alongside his or her non-disabled peers and form early relationships, social development and play. Harris (2000) argues on the basis of a methodological critique of the evidence for parental influence that the social context matters most, and that there is strong evidence to suggest that identification with a peer group is at least as important to young children's socialization as the influence of their parents.

Inclusion at school age: primary and secondary

As children with learning difficulties move on into school, most families will look first to their local primary school. However, the bar is immediately raised; as children grow older, and move into larger schools, with more emphasis on subject learning, inclusion can become more problematic (Frederikson and Cline, 2002: ch. 9). Secondary education is generally considered a far more difficult context for inclusion than primary education, and this is supported for instance by research about the factors promoting inclusion of young people with autistic spectrum disorders in mainstream secondary schools (Osborne and Reed, 2011). Unsurprisingly, this factor analysis showed that those in schools with larger numbers of children with SEN felt more settled than where an isolated child with learning difficulties was included in a mainstream setting.

An official report by the school inspection agency (Ofsted, 2004) reported that the numbers of special school places in England and Wales had remained constant since 1999, although there was considerable variation noted across different local authority areas. Commitment to mainstream education in a local area can therefore make a big difference to the progress of inclusion. The same inspection body commissioned a comprehensive review, including 345 case studies of individual children, and reported that: 'no one model of educational support – such as special schools, full inclusion in mainstream provision, or specialist units co-located with mainstream settings – systematically worked better than any other' (Ofsted, 2010: 11).

There can be systemic problems for learners who need extra support, who may have a lower starting level than the majority of their peers, and who make slower progress through the key stages. It is clearly against the best interests of a school to have too many children with SEN, for instance, if the school is then held responsible for the eventual low outcomes, and is then deemed to be a 'failing school'. Multi-site case studies by Black-Hawkins (2010) found that headteachers and staff often resist the concept of inclusion, drawing on a number of assumptions about the relationship between inclusion and achievement. The drive for standards and measurable outcome targets has led to a competitive system, in which schools are pitted against each other in a quasi-market place, as Barton has also argued (2003: 61). Others support this position:

> The government faced the 150-year-old dilemma over the costs of educating young people who might not be economically profitable to society and who did not fit into a human capital equation. (Tomlinson, 2005: 104)

Inclusive education practices also raise the issue of other students' attitudes. Bullying and harassment are considered major problems in the literature (Mepham, 2010), but are not uniquely associated with inclusive education. On the basis of evidence from 507 children gathered through workshops and an accessible survey, Mepham argues that inclusion of disabled children in mainstream society will reduce their vulnerability to bullying and abuse (2010: 19). Young disabled people in Bristol produced a DVD about their experiences of bullying (see 'Resources' at end of chapter) in which they stress that their experiences are more about isolation, feeling different and other children's misunderstandings.

Paradoxically, then, there are still many proponents of the need for special education. Inspection results in 2010 (Ofsted, 2010) showed very favourable outcomes for special educational establishments, and research has shown no clear support for the positive academic or social effects of either 'inclusion in mainstream' or special schooling (Lindsay, 2007). Therefore, the arguments for mainstream inclusion and specialist provision are still raging in the UK. Recent case studies (Glazzard, 2011) have shown how varied teacher attitudes towards inclusion can coexist within one primary school. Lack of funding, resources and training are frequently cited as barriers, and parents can also be resistant to inclusion. One of the arguments is that pupils with SEN will adversely affect the progress of others. However, a systematic review of evidence about the effect of inclusion on the achievement of *other* mainstream pupils (Kalambouka, 2007) concluded that the majority (81 per cent) of the research studies suggest either neutral or positive effects of including pupils with SEN in mainstream schools.

It is interesting to note that there are also debates in other countries, where inclusive schooling is a norm, supported by governmental legislation. Wendelborg and Tossebro (2010) for instance, describe a longitudinal interpretative study of twenty-six families of disabled children in Norway, where, as they say, the last state-run 'special' school closed in 1992. The sample included at least fifteen children with the labels 'moderate to severe' relative to learning disability. These families reported that their children became gradually less 'included' over the course of their primary school years:

It is the increasing relative gap between children with intellectual disabilities in particular and their peers and the demands of their environment which is the single most striking difference from early to late primary school. (Wendelborg and Tossebro, 2010: 712)

Inclusion in further education

The motivation to develop a social life and make friends is what often drives young people to seek further and higher education, on leaving school. Young people with learning disabilities are no different, and the move into a further education (FE) course is often at least partly about keeping or developing friendships and being included in a social environment (Everitt and Williams, 2007; Doughty and Allan, 2008). Tomlinson (1996) introduced the term that is still current in 2012 in English colleges, 'students with learning difficulties and/or disabilities', a term which included not only those with 'learning difficulties' in the sense of 'special educational needs' but anyone who may need support in college to achieve their educational goals. From the start, FE colleges strove to provide not only specialist courses, but also opportunities to support students with learning difficulties in accessing the full range of provision throughout the college. Because support funding followed the individual student, it was relatively easy to plan appropriate support for a particular student to achieve their own goals, and colleges in the 1980s and 1990s in the UK strove to develop cross-college approaches, where all staff had the skills to include students with learning difficulties (Sutcliffe, 1992).

In the early years of the twenty-first century, there have been many policy initiatives to review and improve provision in the FE sector. *Through Inclusion to Excellence* (LSC, 2005) and *Learning for Living and Work* (LSC, 2006) promote certain key priorities for students with learning difficulties and/or disabilities:

- increased access to high-quality provision;
- improvements in quality of teaching and learning;
- increased participation in learning;
- increased economic participation;
- increased social inclusion; and
- increased levels of attainment.

However, putting these principles into practice is not always easy. For instance, 'increased economic participation and social inclusion' imply that one central task for FE is to help students move on into paid work. Jacobsen (2002) found that students with learning disabilities needed particular support and guidance in order to find appropriate routes into employment and further learning, after their college courses had finished. Students with learning disabilities often needed more direct, practical experience of work, and a 'supported employment' service in order to move into paid employment (see Chapter 10, pp. 182–4). Beyer *et al.* (2004), as well as more recent work (Watson *et al.*, 2006), have investigated the links between education and employment opportunities. The key ingredients for success appear to be good individual vocational profiling; strong work-based learning (including targeted work experience); good links with local employers, and ongoing support for employees, including 'natural' supports in the workplace. FE providers are in a good position to provide at least part of this package, and inclusive research at Cornwall People First (CPF, 2012) found that FE college courses can successfully provide direct job coaching (see also Chapter 10).

Despite the raft of interest in policy and practice terms, there has been sparse research over the decade since 2000 to show how these students are faring. Inspection of provision for students with SEN has included the FE sector, and the 2010 report distinguished between those students who were enrolled on mainstream courses, and those on specially designed courses (studying what is known as a 'pre-entry' or 'entry' level curriculum). In the latter type of provision, assessment of students was found to be 'variable', leading to less effective support.

Further, a local qualitative study in the south-west of England (Everitt *et al.*, 2007) highlighted some problems in social inclusion within colleges, with students with learning difficulties effectively segregated in specialist enclaves, and remaining isolated from mainstream students. This is a picture also reflected in a review of the literature:

> Students with severe learning difficulties are generally welcomed, but as a hidden minority; are allocated to their own classrooms, often following non-accredited programmes; and are separated from the higher profile courses offered by the institution. (Wright, 2006: 36)

There are also notable gaps in provision for those with more profound and complex needs, as well as students with autism, a point reiterated in the most recent inspection report (Ofsted, 2010). Meanwhile, a current Ph.D. study (Fox, 2012) is examining the communication needs of students with learning disabilities, and how these are met within the context of an FE college. If inclusion is to be successful, then a whole college approach must be taken, where all staff and facilities are part of the picture.

Inclusion in practice

Moving towards a more inclusive system

This book follows the position that it is segregated, not inclusive, provision which should have to be justified. Inclusion is a right, and a norm. However, in order to get it right, systemic changes may be needed at a number of levels. One of the keys to finding a way forward is to return to some reflection on the model underpinning education for young people with learning difficulties. All too often, the child is seen as the problem, as identified by Diez (2010) in Spain. 'Medical model' thinking leads professionals to locate within-child deficits, and to supply special programmes and supports to address those deficits. By contrast, social model thinking leads to more systemic solutions, where the task becomes about overcoming the barriers placed in the way of disabled children in a school system that is premised on normalcy and achievement (Wendelborg and Tossebro, 2010; Armstrong and Barton, 2008).

In practice, as argued earlier in this chapter, it is often necessary to consider a relational model, which reflects both the child's intrinsic needs and the environment. What do these models look like in practice? Weddell (2008) neatly reviews progress in making systemic changes, and he groups these under four headings. These are: curriculum, pedagogy, structure of schooling and local authorities. He argues that we could frequently be accused of 'patching up' a system which is inherently non inclusive. However, Weddell (2008) gives some recent examples of progress and systemic change. Table 4.1 outlines some of these.

There are many dilemmas underlying these changes, and often contradictions in policy and practice that undermine the moves towards inclusion. As Weddell (2008) argues, what is needed is 'flexibility' in the system, but this flexibility has to be based on changes that are about the whole education system, and not just solutions that patch up the problem at an individual level. At FE level, for instance, personal portfolios with photos and personal planning information can be developed with individual students, but will only have an effect on inclusion within the whole college, with: (a) commitment from senior management; (b) including other agencies in annual review process for each student; (c) training for trainers on advocacy; (d) timing allowed for this work for college staff (not an addition to normal teaching timetable) (Jacobsen, 2005).

Table 4.1	Systemic changes for school inclusion	
	Systemic changes	**'Patching-up' initiatives**
Curriculum	'Opening Minds' curriculum: a major focus on learning, citizenship, relating to people, managing situations, managing people: now being piloted.	Children with SEN are disapplied from the requirements of standardized testing (SATs)
Pedagogy	'Personalized learning for all': involvement of experts to advise and work with teachers – e.g. SENCo services from outside the school.	'Personalized learning' introduced without sufficient training.
Structure of schooling	Dividing the teaching day into two long teaching periods – to enable flexible arrangements of team teaching, small groups, individual learning.	Paying for coaching outside school for children.
Local authorities	Development of children's trusts within local authorities – aimed at bringing education, health, social services together within one organization.	Articulate parents fight for the rights of their own child's statement of SEN to be met.

Source: based on Weddell, 2008

Partnerships with parents

Partnership is at the heart of ensuring a successful educational experience for all those children who experience SEN, at any stage of their school career. The success stories about children with severe learning difficulties are all to do with a range of professionals, as well as parents, working together to achieve change. This can be done within a person-centred planning (PCP) framework, where those close to the child can help to outline clearly the personality, strengths and goals of the individual child. PCP methods are explored in more depth in Chapter 7.

A parent of a teenager with Autism Spectrum Disorder (ASD) in the UK, who has co-taught on an M.Sc. programme at the University of Bristol commented that the transition to secondary education was the most difficult stage for her son. However, she (the parent) knew very well what strategies would work, and the kind of learning style her son favoured. For instance, in learning about abstract concepts in geography, it was far more effective for him to learn from practical experiences and from multisensory approaches. Because parents have supported their children since birth, they will know the fine detail about 'what works', which might be very different for every child.

In order for children like this to be included effectively, there must be open and transparent discussion between family, school and child. Much depends on systems that the school can set up for communicating with parents, and these will include:

- home school diaries;
- email contact with parents;
- face-to-face meetings; and
- a policy of open visits, or specified times for informal coffee mornings with parents.

Often, this entails breaking down the traditional barriers of privacy surrounding the individual teacher in their classroom; successful and flexible 'personalized learning' requires a team teaching approach, and sensitive deployment of learning support resources.

Professional practices

Responses to meeting the needs of children with SEN will differ in various contexts. Ainscow (1999) for instance, found situations in developing countries where very few resources were available to support inclusion, but where children with additional needs were nevertheless within ordinary classrooms, sometimes with pupil numbers in the area of 70 or 80 per class. Those who were experiencing difficulties in learning or in keeping up with the lesson would rely on other pupils to repeat and revise the lesson with them, after the end of the class.

In the UK, one of the main strategies for supporting children with SEN in mainstream classrooms is the use of teaching assistants (TAs), sometimes also called learning support assistants (LSAs). Despite their deployment in many countries, such as the USA, Giangreco (2010) points out that there is very little evidence or theory behind their role. Farrell *et al.* (2010) conducted a systematic review of research in this field, and found that targeted interventions by LSAs resulted in improved standards, whereas more general LSA work in whole class support 'may not have a positive impact on the achievement of all pupils' (Farrell *et al.*, 2010: 435). Essentially, using learning support assistants involves putting another adult in the classroom, to ensure that one or more of the children with SEN receive the attention and level of teaching which they need. However, the problem in deploying LSAs is that they become attached to an individual child, thus:

1. becoming effectively the teacher for that child;
2. standing as a barrier between that child and the actual teacher; and
3. preventing social interaction between the target child and others in the classroom.

These are multiple and interacting problems here. It is easy for the teacher to think that the child with SEN is effectively catered for because she or he has their own support in place. This situation is known in the trade as the 'velcro-LSA', where the child can become very dependent on their own individual support worker, and in fact will respond by demonstrating 'learned helplessness', a concept adapted from the field of mental health (Seligman, 1975), in which an individual learns a passive form of behaviour. By contrast, an LSA can be considered to be part of the teaching team, and may be far more effectively used to support the whole teaching situation, allowing greater flexibility to meet all the children's needs. That is likely to promote better inclusion, despite the findings above from Farrell's review, that this practice does not always promote better achievement. Perhaps the solution lies in good training and team work, as in the following 'win-win' example:

> In a large secondary comprehensive school, an LSA was observed, who was supporting a science teacher, with a number of children with significant learning difficulties – about 4 or 5 out of a class of 30. As the lesson was being introduced, it was about to be a science practical – the teacher was talking at the front, talking about the equipment that was going to be needed. The LSA was behind him at the whiteboard, writing it clearly – 'bunsen burner' and drawing the Bunsen burner. And putting it as '1' because it is the first thing they need to collect, then the beaker and so on. It was team work, and that was obviously essential for the 4 or 5 children who she was supporting, but it was also incredibly useful for all the other children – who may have specific learning difficulties, everybody in fact. But it was also maximizing the use of that LSA, and seeing that person as supporting the whole teaching that was going on in the class; she was not seen as velcroed to the particular children she was supporting.

The role of learning support assistants is vital, and recognized also in other EU countries, such as Ireland (Abbott *et al.*, 2011). This research found that learning support assistants were under-qualified in Ireland, and all parties felt that they were in need of further training. The LSA was often the person left to cope with any challenging behaviour or disruption in school. These are sensitive tasks, and it is vital that the professional status and training of the LSA matches the role (see also Brandon and Charlton, 2011; Jones, 2010).

Tackling bullying

The philosophy of inclusive education can sound like thin rhetoric when children and families are concerned about harassment and discrimination. Bullying can happen within any educational context. One clear indication from research is that it is not enough simply to provide an 'inclusive culture'; bullying has to be tackled proactively and action taken to promote open communication about bullying and to ensure that individual incidents are tackled. Research about bullying at international level has been concerned to identify the predictors, so that preventative action can effectively be taken. For instance, a systematic review, identifying 153 studies about bullying, found that:

> To the extent that aggression and bullying are part of the normative context of development, it may be that only interventions addressing individual and contextual factors simultaneously will evidence positive effects. (Cook *et al.*, 2010: 80)

Bullying can be a problem for many young people in school, not just those with learning difficulties, and Hartas and Lindsay (2011) demonstrate clearly that young people themselves can contribute useful suggestions for tackling bullying; in their study, for instance, children suggested direct action, including a greater emphasis on involving parents of bullies.

At FE level, some good practice initiatives to prevent bullying and ensure greater cohesion between all students were also highlighted by colleges in Everitt *et al.* (2007). The particular initiatives were:

- A peer advocacy scheme with experienced students visiting new applicants at home.
- The use of visual means of recording experiences at introductory taster days in college.
- Organization of cross-college events, which students with learning disabilities can sometimes lead.

Including students' voices

There are numerous policy imperatives to listen to the voices of learners, at international and at national level. The right for children to be heard is included in the UN Convention on the Rights of People with Disabilities (Article 7.3), which states that: 'Parties shall ensure that children with disabilities have the right to express their views freely on all matters affecting them.' In England, the Education Act 2002 placed a duty on schools to consult with pupils about decisions that affect them, and the Green Paper *Every Child Matters* emphasized children's partic-ipation in developing policies and services (DfES, 2003). As Hartas and Lindsay (2011: 129–30) argue, listening to young people can enhance educational services, and build the capacity for individual pupils to feel a sense of ownership within the school.

Instead of simply engaging with a single student about their own education, this type of listening is about encouraging young disabled people to develop a collective voice, so that they can have active representation in the debates about inclusive schooling.

Some ideas emerge from recent work in which young people have been included more actively within development projects, production of materials, and within research. The following list gives some examples:

- Learners need time and support to be able to develop the self-confidence to speak up. The skills of self-advocacy can become a more central part of the curriculum for all learners (see resource list at end of chapter).
- Children and young people can be enabled to move from individual positions towards a more 'collective' voice, by enabling them to have their own organi-zation for example, a group for young disabled people in Bristol called the Listening Partnership.
- Young people can be included as researchers. Kellett (2011) reports on research undertaken by a group of young people with learning difficulties, showing how they too can participate and have a voice.

Further, it is possible to seek views from children beyond their own individual goals, as Whitehurst (2006) did, by devising creative methods in which a group of children with complex needs were offered the chance to experience an inclusive drama production with 'mainstream' children, and were then asked about their reactions:

> Children are children first – it is their right and our obligation to ensure that when we talk about inclusion we take their views into account.
> (Whitehurst, 2006: 60)

Jacobsen (2005) reports on similar initiatives at FE level, where students with learning difficulties created dramas and videos to illustrate how person-centred planning (see Chapter 7) can be used in FE.

Recent work by Davies *et al.* (2012) has included young people with learning disabilities as researchers, to talk with others and analyse what matters to those who are included in mainstream education. The social aspects of being included loomed large for these youngsters, who were nonetheless able to suggest several practical solutions to their schools. Nilholm and Alm (2010) in the context of a Swedish inclusive classroom, attempted to define some methods to capture the complexity of all children's experiences, those with disabilities and their non-disabled classmates. The point of view of the children themselves was central to this study, and three main criteria of inclusion were used: (a) differences being viewed as ordinary; (b) all students being part of the social community of the classroom; and (c) all students being part of the learning community of the classroom (Nilholm and Alm, 2010: 243). These Swedish researchers found that interviews and children's poems gave a more complex picture of inclusion than a simple survey, and a poem from that study in Sweden is included in the words of students with learning difficulties with which this chapter started:

I am never alone, never feel that way,
even though the others seem to think so.
They don't really know what I feel.

Conclusion: what has educational inclusion achieved?

Inclusion as a policy goal has been supported, as seen in this chapter, by repeated government strategies and practice initiatives in England, since the early 1990s. How has it fared, in bringing about change? There has been considerable progress over that period, and it is far more likely now for a child with learning disabilities to be offered a place in a mainstream school than it was in 1992, with 60 per cent of children with statements of SEN now educated in the mainstream. However, over that period there has also been a good deal of debate about what is actually meant by inclusion, with the pendulum now swinging towards the notion of an inclusive system, rather than inclusive locations. Therefore, it could be argued that the policy concept of 'inclusion' has been enlarged and reshaped, very much in line with the wider view of education as a function of society. However, there are also potential problems here with a system that retreats from pursuing inclusion, simply because of a lack of skills, resources or supports for children with learning difficulties. It could be argued therefore that the ideals of an inclusive education system will never be achieved until education is really seen as a universal *entitlement* rather than a competitive system where one school is set against another.

Research about inclusion, as summarized in this chapter, has largely failed to come up with robust quantitative evidence about the outcomes of locational inclusion; however, interpretative studies have helped to understand the obstacles faced by mainstream schools, including academic targets and teacher attitudes. In countries other than the UK, inclusion in mainstream education also appears to become more difficult to achieve as children become older, and move into secondary education. However, action research and evaluation of interventions are all important in underlining both the barriers to inclusion, but also some possible solutions. This chapter has highlighted particularly the importance of taking a systemic view of inclusion, and therefore the importance of systemic thinking about the changes that need to be made. For instance, where teaching assistants are used in more collaborative fashion, then all children can benefit.

Although the inclusion debate is far from resolved, children with learning difficulties in England have gained increasing rights over the past twenty years to an education which meets their own needs, alongside their peers. There are practical ways in which inclusion can be promoted, through partnership work with parents, ensuring sufficient support and training are delivered to all staff, including teaching assistants, including children themselves in the debates, and by tackling some of the difficulties which children tell us they face – such as bullying. However, inclusion is not just something that is 'done' to children with learning difficulties. A system that is truly inclusive will bring benefits to all pupils, those with special educational needs, as well as all others.

Reflection exercises

1. 'Molly's' story is an amalgam of several examples and stories told by young people with learning difficulties, offered here to promote reflection on the points in this chapter.

   Molly was a young girl aged 11, who had been in a special unit attached to a mainstream primary school. Her move to a large, inner-city comprehensive school provoked some anxieties amongst the staff, who asked the educational psychologist to go in and provide some training. The main issue was that Molly had Down's syndrome, and so had a recognizable impairment. Staff were unsure what they could expect from Molly, or whether they needed to take account of her limitations. The trainer told them quite the opposite: that they needed to fight against lowered expectations, and give Molly the opportunity to show what she could do. In terms of health and safety, Molly was at first allocated a teaching assistant to support her during break times. However, Molly herself kept running away, saying she did not want the TA to be listening to what she said to her friends. During the first year at school, Molly's parents were regularly invited in, and had an email link with school staff to discuss any issues which arose. However, after just one term, her parents reported not only that Molly was surviving in school, but that she had made a tremendous amount of progress socially.

2. Consider how all staff in a school can become motivated to contribute to change, and to develop their confidence in finding solutions to include a student such as Molly.

3. Review what research has shown about the barriers faced by children with learning difficulties, and work out what problems might be expected to face Molly in her progress through secondary school. Discuss with others how these might be tackled, and how different professionals may contribute to joint working in supporting Molly.

4. What does inclusion mean, and is it still a useful word in the development of educational policy? It may be most revealing to think about this by asking some young people with and without learning difficulties, who have current or recent experience as school students.

Suggested further resources

1. Young disabled people made an 'animation' video about inclusion: Fleming Fulton School: Inclusion DVD is available (from 10 March 2012) at: www.youtube.com/user/flemingfultonbelfast/feed

2. The Alliance for Inclusive Education has useful resources, including online access to their magazine, 'Inclusion Now' which is packed with information and examples: www.allfie.org.uk

3. There are useful books, free to download about personal planning and a workbook for young people with learning disabilities *My Kind of a Future*, available from the Foundation for People with Learning Disabilities at:

http://learningdisabilities.org.uk/publications/

Teachers' TV has developed videos that are free to download and use for discussion, and for examples of inclusion. They are now available at www.tes.co.uk. Follow the links to 'Teachers' TV' and 'Special Needs'.

5 Partnership with Families

Families have always been central to the lives of people with learning disabilities, at all ages. Although not all people with learning disabilities have support from their families, nevertheless for many it is commonly accepted that family members are the basis onto which other support is built. Family members are there because they love and care for their relative with learning disabilities, and without them the social care system in the UK, and in other countries, would not be able to function. Since they have such an important role, it is vital that families are supported to work in partnership with professionals. While the 'Voices of Experience' boxes in other chapters exclusively belong to people with learning disabilities, this chapter foregrounds mainly the voices of parents and families.

Key points summary:

- Families are very important for people with learning disabilities, often throughout their lives.
- Parents have a right to support, information and advice from the first years of their child's life. Parents of children with learning disabilities say they need services to work together better.
- Parents should be partners, along with professionals, in supporting their relative with learning disabilities. People who are partners share the same goal, but may have different roles in getting there.
- Families are all different. Some end up taking on big jobs in managing the services for their relative with learning disabilities, while others do not wish to or may not have the need to do that. There are also some people with learning disabilities who have had problems with their families.
- Paid staff and other professionals need to work together as equals with families. It is important for all of them to listen to what the person with learning disabilities wants, and what may work best for that person.

Introduction and overview

 Voice of Experience

> My mother ... looked for the good in me, she treated me as any other child would be treated. She got joy out of me as she did with all her other children. And when there were stories in the family they were all about the good things that we remembered. My mum had prevented the first separation of my life from society. But she had gone beyond this. She had made a commitment to place me in society where I belonged just like everybody else.
>
> *Source*: Anya Souza, in Souza with Ramcharan, 1997: 5

When a learning disability is diagnosed, it generally brings in its wake offers of support from professionals and services. Much of this is very necessary and there have been many steps forward in providing timely support to families in recent years in the UK. This chapter will explore that support from the viewpoint of families themselves. The role of parents and families in the lives of people with learning disabilities does not stop when their child reaches the age of 18, and that was also true for Anya Souza, whose comments opened this chapter. Over the last century, families have continued to be central to learning disability support and indeed in many countries, families are the only option in terms of support and care for their relative with learning disabilities. In Western countries there have been traditions of provided services such as day centres and residential homes. However, even in the UK, with the moves towards personalized services, family carers in general (over all impairment groups) have been shown to save the state as much as £87 billion, through their unpaid labour (Buckner and Yeandle, 2007). For many reasons, therefore, this chapter should be considered a central one in the current book.

Community care legislation in England has recognized the rights of carers and family members in recent years, with a series of Acts of Parliament, introducing legislation which gives carers a right to have their own needs assessed and considered. The major pieces of English legislation relating to carers' needs, which build on each other, are summarized in Box 5.1. (See also Box 7.1 in Chapter 7 for transition policies.)

Families are diverse, and do not all fit one model. Some are prepared and able to tackle official systems, and devote massive amounts of time and energy to the support of their son or daughter, well into their adulthood, as Anya Souza's mother did (see box above). Others, inevitably, will not be prepared or will not have the resources to do this. However, there is an urgent need to ensure that all families are well supported and valued, so that they can continue to contribute, in the way that they wish, to the lives of their son or daughter with learning disabilities. That is the reason for linking the discussion of families in this chapter with the key concept of partnership.

Box 5.1	Legislation that affects families of people with learning disabilities

Carers (Recognition and Services) Act 1995

This act gave carers important new rights and a clear legal status. Individuals who provide or intend to provide a substantial amount of care on a regular basis are entitled to request (at the time the person they care for is being assessed for community care services), an assessment of their ability to care and to continue caring. Although local authorities had to take account of the 'results of this assessment', however, they were still only able to provide services directly to the person with learning disabilities, until the ...

Carers and Disabled Children Act 2000

- gave local councils mandatory duties to support carers by providing services to carers directly;
- empowered local authorities to make direct payments to carers; and
- enabled councils to support flexibility in provision of short breaks through the short break voucher scheme.

Carers (Equal Opportunities) Act 2004

- placed a duty on councils to inform carers, in certain circumstances, of their right to an assessment of their needs;
- provided that when assessing a carer's needs, councils must take into account whether the carer works or wishes to work, undertakes or wishes to undertake education, training or leisure activities; and
- facilitated cooperation between authorities in relation to the provision of services that are relevant to carers.

Work and Families Act 2006

This extended the right to request flexible working to employees who care for adults. This built on the introduction (through the Employment Act 2002) of the right to request flexible working for parents of children under the age of 6 (or 18 if the child is disabled).

The following section will explore some theoretical points about partnership working, as well as information about some of the efforts to establish partnerships with parents and families of people with learning disabilities. Evidence from research and accounts by family members themselves, however, often differ from the policy goals reflected above. As explored in this chapter, research evidence reveals that some families face extreme stress (Mansell and Wilson, 2010), the negative socio-economic consequences of caring (Burton-Smith *et al.*, 2009), as well as disempowerment and sometimes distrust from professionals. Conflicts between professionals and families can occur because of safeguarding concerns, and author- ities sometimes step in to protect the best interests of the relative with learning disabilities (Williams *et al.*, 2012). Nevertheless, the key message from most fami- lies is that they want services and supports to be right for their relative with learn- ing disabilities; that is the most important goal, and in theory will provide the basis for a fruitful partnership. This chapter will therefore set out some of the evidence for developing partnership working with families, and the concluding sections particularly reflect on partnership work that keeps the balance right, through a joint focus on the needs and wishes of the person with learning disabilities.

Key policy concept: partnership

What is partnership?

'Partnership' is a marked word in policy – it is invoked precisely in order to contrast with other, less favourable ways of working. Partnership is often flagged as a key goal precisely when there are underlying structural disincentives to joint work, as in health and social care partnerships (Bridgen and Lewis, 1999). If people are not working in partnership, they are working in isolation, in competi- tion, or sometimes at loggerheads, with each other. Moreover, if partnership working between professionals is difficult to achieve, then meaningful partner- ships between professionals and families are even harder to attain. It has been claimed that 'constant practical difficulties with making partnership work and misunderstandings about the meaning of partnership between families and profes- sionals have, in many cases, devalued its principle' (Lacey, 2001: 135).

Most definitions of partnership include joint work towards shared goals, albeit with different roles for each partner. The following features of partnership work- ing underpin policy, and are here applied to working in partnership with families:

- **Sharing of goals**: for instance, parents who manage support services for their adult son or daughter with learning disabilities may share the same goals with the local authority services – to ensure that their offspring have support to meet their needs, to keep safe and so on. However, parents and local authority staff may have different roles within the shared partnership.
- **Equality**: in England, since 2001, local social services departments have set up partnership boards, to discuss and develop learning disability services. Both family carers and people with learning disabilities themselves are invited onto these boards, in order to discuss matters to do with services, in theory on an equal basis with local authority managers (Fyson and Fox, 2008).
- **Person-centredness**: 'person-centred' partnerships imply that the individual with learning disabilities remains the focus, and in control of the partnership work going on around him or her. In good person-centred planning (see Chapter 7), this is essentially what happens for the individual person with learning disabilities.

Of course, these features of good partnership working are not always apparent. In practice, there are many threats, and it is easy for 'partnership' to become yet another buzzword, representing nothing more than warm feelings. It may be useful therefore to consider the different levels of partnership for professional working, and to see whether and how they could apply to working in partnership with parents and families. Box 5.2 illustrates this type of layered model, where progress is assumed to be made towards joint working.

Box 5.2	**Different levels on the continuum of 'joined up working'**
No partnership	Learning Disability services set up with no regard to the parent or family of the disabled person.
Level one: cooperation	Services and families work together toward consistent goals and complementary services.
Level two: collaboration	Families help services to plan ahead and address issues of overlap, duplication and gaps in service provision towards common outcomes
Level three: coordination	Families and services work together in a planned and systematic manner towards shared and agreed goals

Source: based on Frost, 2005; see also Lacey, 2001: 10–11

The terms of partnership from the parental perspective

Partnership often means work. Parents in the UK are expected not only to receive services, but also to contribute to local service provision and to participate in local decision making. For instance, Blair (2009) described a London based group of parents, who contributed to education of health and social care professionals. Similarly, a local multi-agency steering group is normally needed to plan and manage the introduction of support for disabled children in the early years. Such groups should include parents, and the 'Change for Children' programme urges local managers to consider 'how to sustain the participation of families in planning and service development initiatives over time'.

Nevertheless, these partnerships may not always be based on an equal relationship. Rix and Paige-Smith (2008) carried out a study with parents of young children with learning disabilities, and found that their participation in early years interventions often depended on their acceptance of the professional terms of the intervention. Effectively, they were asked to take up strong roles as agents for change in their children's development, but to do that on the terms of the professional structures around them. Interestingly, several parents involved in that study had taken on professional roles themselves, in leading parent support groups or volunteering in different ways.

Partnership as a concept is clearly not a panacea. Instead, it has to be differentiated, and applied in a way that both empowers families, but also protects and honours the rights of people with learning disabilities when that is needed. Effectively, this type of partnership is a three-way affair, with people with learning disabilities at the centre. Achieving that centrality in practice however appears to be harder in some cases than others, and certainly requires skills and commitment on the part of parents and family carers. This chapter therefore turns next to a summary of some of the research about families of people with learning disabilities, with a focus on their own perspectives.

Research evidence about families of people with learning disabilities

Experience of having a baby with a learning disability

Voice of Experience

There were changes, leaps and bounds with Jack. Suddenly when he started recognizing people, with his gargle. And I thought: 'Wow' and he had favourites, a couple of carers. So you knew that he wasn't just a care package, there was a person in there.

(Reproduced with kind permission of a parent of baby with complex needs; personal communication, 2009)

The 'diagnosis' of learning disability may be experienced in very different ways, according to the stage at which it happens, the particular professionals involved and the parents' own prior knowledge (Bostrom *et al.*, 2010). Therefore parents speak of some very different experiences of being told about their child's learning disability, as is evident from the examples in Rolph *et al.'s* (2005) narrative research with families, are included in the Voices of Experience box on page 77.

As the opening quotation in this section indicates, parents will recognize the unique personality of each disabled child, just as with any child. Even a very severely disabled infant is more than 'just a care package'. However, for many parents, the problems come to dominate that relationship, particularly when they do not have a diagnosis. A parent from the USA, who wrote of her experiences (Foster-Galasso, 2005), says that she actually sought out a diagnosis for her son, because of the problems of which she was aware. She talked about her ambivalent relationship with diagnosis, especially the 'words' that have been used to describe her son (autism, pervasive developmental disorder). On occasions, she writes, these words are ones that the family has deliberately sought out, or used, for specific purposes:

Voices of Experience

'We were left to get on with it'

Then soon she was coming home, they packed her off home with us and that was it, we were left to get on with it. We weren't really told what was wrong with her or anything ... the only explanation we ever really got was that Rachel would be a little bit slow ... I knew nothing about it at all. I just never realised that children could be like that'.

'I discovered what was wrong with him'

I read it all up. I took it upon myself to go to the library and go through all the medical textbooks until I discovered what was wrong with him. I was told when he was nine months. That doesn't seem very long now but at the time it did seem like an eternity.

'We bonded instantly, and loved our beautiful baby'

Negative images portrayed by some of the medical profession: 'they don't suck very well', 'she probably won't talk because she has a big tongue', 'they don't usually live beyond the age of five'. We felt like this was an alien! No one takes it on themselves to predict what will happen in the life of a non-disabled baby.

Whether to use a diagnosis, and if so, which one? A lot depends on the purpose of the conversation or interrogation. Is it a gateway to something we need or not? (Foster-Galasso, 2005: 20)

A word such as 'autism' can push open a 'stuck gate', for instance by providing the reason for a support assistant or aide in school. At other times, however, Foster-Galasso talks of lay reactions to her child's behaviour. When a diagnostic word like 'autistic' comes into play, people cease to treat him like an individual child, and assume he is just 'one of them', part of a group of people who are different and who must be socially avoided.

It is also important to remember the complex and differentiated picture of cultural differences which exist in the UK and elsewhere. For instance, among South Asian families in the UK, the prevalence of learning disabilities is at least twice as high as in other communities (Azmi *et al.*, 1997; Hatton *et al.*, 2004). However, there are many cultural factors which will influence how these families cope with the task of bringing up a disabled child (Skinner and Weisner, 2007). These include the effect of traditional religious beliefs about the cause of impairment, as well as language barriers which compound the lack of understanding of explanations given by medical professionals and others (Hatton *et al.*, 2010). An action research study by Raghavan *et al.* (2005) found that South Asian families were reluctant to take up state-provided services for a number of reasons, but were not necessarily replacing that by support from their own communities. Therefore, there is a special need to pay attention to communication, information and support that is culturally appropriate for minority community families, who may be doubly disadvantaged.

In all cultural and ethnic groups, it is of course possible for babies to be born who have very complex health care needs, and due to technological advances in perinatal health care, these babies are increasingly likely to survive for longer periods. Family members in these instances are faced with the sudden necessity to learn and apply skills relating to health, well-being and survival for their disabled child, and Dawkins (2009) describes her own role in providing care for her son with profound and multiple learning disabilities, claiming that 60 per cent of parents in her situation spend more than ten hours a day on basic physical care. One particular case was mentioned in Chapter 3, which related to a baby we called 'Jack'. For Jack's parents, their infant was first and foremost a human being with a unique personality, and this is how they wanted him to be treated by health professionals. The problems they experienced continued even after their baby was at home with them. They were supported by carers on four nights a week, and a few hours during the day. While this was absolutely necessary for their survival as a family, they could see again the blinkered view the carers had of Jack as a unique individual:

Voice of Experience

All the carers were very good, but they were trained. To them, he was a care package, and they had to write miles and miles of useless rubbish. And nobody ever looked at it. I've got a whole cupboard full of it. It wasn't necessary, and it was wasting time. Most of them got into that kind of work because they wanted to interact, and have more of an impact and friendship, and see a development. But this was so clinical. It concentrated on his needs, and not who he was.

(Reproduced with kind permission of a parent of baby with complex needs; personal communication, 2009)

The central message that emerged from Jack's story was the need to look beyond the health needs, even when there were such complex and multiple problems. In fact, the greater and more profound the learning disability, the more it is necessary to find ways to engage with the child himself. Indeed, that is a constant in the life of many people with learning disabilities: Mansell (2010) emphasized the same need to recognize the individual's personality, in adults with profound and multiple learning disabilities.

Parents' relationship with childhood professionals

 Voice of Experience

When they're young, 2 or 3, you know you're going to have your health visitor there, you know you're going to be doing all that stuff. But I suppose at that point, when they would normally be going away, when they could see you doing things right, and you wouldn't see them as much, they were around for longer and longer. And that's what made it different I think.

(Reproduced with kind permission of the parent of a man with complex needs; personal communication, 2010)

The introduction of professional services into private family life is all too often experienced both as an intrusion and a threat. Attempts to provide support to disabled children and to their parents can often be the first signal to them that their life is going to be different from that of other families. The quotation above relates to a period of time some twenty or more years ago. Yet similar stories can still be heard from parents of young people with learning disabilities, including those with babies who have multiple and complex health needs (Townsley *et al.*, 2004).

In the UK and other Western countries, when a child is diagnosed as having a learning disability, or any significant or complex impairment, the family may have 'services' or visits from a wide range of professionals, such as the following:

- health visitor;
- early years support worker;
- portage educator;
- home child carer; and
- speech and language therapist.

The English Department for Children, Schools and Families provides a booklet called 'People you may meet', which gives definitions of the roles of 46 workers who may come into contact with families of children with special needs or disabilities (DCSF, 2007c). Lacey (2001: 7–8) lists 43 specialist agencies that may have responsibility for a child with learning disabilities, from the health, social care, education and voluntary sectors. Compared with other parents, families of children with learning disabilities soon start to live extremely complex lives, being expected to absorb new information about how to support their child's development, and also to navigate their way through a vast network of supports. It is for this reason that families say they are desperately in need of some coordination and family-centred support (Townsley *et al.*, 2004). This is what the UK government is now trying to achieve, and some of these initiatives will be highlighted in the following section of this chapter.

School entry is seen by all parents as a major step change in their relationship with those outside the family. School–parent partnerships are crucial, but especially so for parents of children with learning disabilities. As mentioned, their child may well have already experienced developmental programmes, input from therapists, and family-centred advice. However, at school age, it is the education authority and the teacher who takes over that responsibility. Unfortunately, parents do not always feel empowered by that relationship. Hornby and Ravleen (2011) for instance analyse the barriers that exist between family and school for all parents, at four different levels: that of the parent and family, the child, the relationship between parent and teacher, and finally at the level of society. These barriers can be magnified in the case of children with learning disabilities, unless schools recognize the wealth of experience and expertise the parent has already built up by the time their child reaches school age. In some cases, that recognition can and does happen, as parents themselves become more empowered to speak up. Langan (2011) argues on the basis of a review of parental accounts that collaborative partnerships have become more frequent since the early 2000s in relation to children with autism and severe learning disabilities, since parental activism has moved the view of autism away from a 'disease' model and towards an understanding of autistic diversity. Narratives and models based on individual families' experiences predominate in this literature. More research is needed, however, to explore the extent to which these shared values and understandings can make a difference to families' experiences.

Educational and social services rightly focus on the child. Parents are partners in that focus, and as seen in Chapter 4, they are vital in supporting and enabling their child to develop. However, they too need support, in order to maintain their role. Repeated research studies based on interviews and focus groups (e.g. Brown *et al.*, 2011 in Scotland; Caples and Sweeney 2011 in Ireland) have found that parents' needs for short break services and supports were not being met. Nevertheless, 23 families of children who had severe challenging behaviour reported that their lives were far more manageable when respite care and specialized day support services were available (Brown *et al.*, 2011). Ways forward will be explored further in the following section.

Advocacy roles of family carers

The relationship between the disabled people's movement in general, and groups representing parents and carers, has not always been an easy one. People with learning disabilities themselves, particularly those who have developed a collective voice through self-advocacy organizations, may not want families to speak for them. Research that has examined the issues of conflicting views within the family has largely concluded that these fears are unfounded (Williams and Robinson, 2001a), although analysis of naturally occurring encounters involving family members reveals that the voice of the parent often takes precedence over the voice of young people with learning disabilities (Pilnick *et al.*, 2011). It is important therefore to remember the fine line between advocating for someone else's rights, and dominating that person's own voice.

Nevertheless, all parents are advocates for their children, in the sense that they speak for them in the early years, and defend their 'best interests', and there is a special sense in which the voice of the parent is identified with the interests of their child with learning disabilities, as Souza very movingly expressed in the opening comments in this chapter. Cole (2005) for instance interviewed six teachers who were also mothers of youngsters with learning disabilities. They articulated the very close way in which a parent becomes allied with the interests of their disabled child:

> **Voice of Experience**
>
> Often it really is the parents. They (the authorities) are accountable to money, not to your child. My responsibility is to be accountable for my son.
>
> (parent, in Cole, 2005: 337)

The reason that parents often become such forceful advocates is precisely because of their children's needs for support, and the frequent problems they encounter in ensuring those needs are met. Runswick-Cole (2007) analysed the stories of parents as advocates for their children at Special Educational Needs tribunals, where a dispute exists between parents and local education authorities (LEAs). Using a narrative inquiry approach, she found that the process of advocating for their child at tribunal had profound effects on the family, not only in terms of their emotional stability, but also on their financial affairs.

This advocacy that parents have to take up does not in the least mean that they see their own children as 'special' or intrinsically different from any other child. Indeed, another striking theme in parents' accounts is their desire for 'normality' and their concern that their child will be seen as 'just normal' (Cole, 2005: 339). This appears to be a cross-cultural theme and for instance Bengali parents of children with learning disabilities in Rao (2006) also argued that their children had normal levels of functioning and intelligence within the family, and they placed great value on being able to achieve social skills and awareness associated with family roles. By contrast, they saw their sons and daughters with learning disabilities being 'pathologized' by educational specialists, who judged them by different yardsticks. Young people with learning disabilities do not have different aspirations, by and large, from other young people. This is also true of their parents: what they want for their children is the same as other parents want – namely happiness, stability, friendships, communication and opportunities to be themselves. However, achieving these things is not always easy for a child with learning disabilities, and so parents find themselves having to fight for inclusive services, and opportunities that other children take for granted. It is parents who have often spearheaded the development of new types of services.

Davies and Morgan (2010) follow through the transition experiences of a group of young people with Down's syndrome, who had person-centred plans, and highlight the role played by their parents as advocates. However, as McCarthy (2010) comments in the same volume, it is problematic that only people with learning disabilities who have these 'pioneer parents' get good services. Solutions for young people and their families must be more readily available for all, and effectively, this must mean changing the systems so that they are not perceived as enemies to progress, but as supports to all families.

The whole family

 Voice of Experience

Having a child that's 'different' sets you apart from other men ... I was so unprepared for the moment (at birth) when I was told my daughter had suffered brain damage ... I needed someone to talk to but there was nobody.

(father, in research by Towers, 2009: preface)

It is important to remember that support for a child with learning disabilities does not just impinge on mothers. Although it is the mother who may often take on the lead role in childcare, a father's experience (as reported above in Towers, 2009) can be ignored, and may be even more difficult because of the societal expectation that men are 'strong' and do not express emotion.

MacDonald and Hastings (2010) conducted a survey of 105 fathers, measuring the extent to which they carried out 'mindful' parenting and the relationship between that measure and their involvement with their child who had learning disabilities. They concluded that these two factors were linked, although it cannot necessarily be inferred that one is a cause of the other. Nevertheless, all this work illustrates both the importance of parents' roles in supporting a child with learning disabilities, and the sensitivity and delicacy of negotiating complex systems of education, health and social care.

Siblings of children with learning disabilities also play important roles, and have corresponding needs for support and recognition; Heller and Arnold (2010) report on a review of 23 relevant studies between 1970 and 2008 about the outcomes for adult siblings of children with learning disabilities. Unsurprisingly, the relationship between siblings tended to be long-lasting, with adult siblings often taking on greater supportive roles as their sibling with a learning disability grew older. However, the psychosocial outcomes for siblings were found to be mixed, and support services for 'young carers' are starting to address the needs that these family members have in childhood and beyond.

From parent to carer

The role of being a parent to someone with a learning disability does not cease when the young person turns eighteen, and officially becomes an adult. Emerson *et al.* (2005) showed that about half of all adults with learning disabilities were still living at home with parents, and a further 12 per cent lived with other relatives. However, from the parents' point of view, being a 'carer' may be something that happens before the magic age of 18 is reached, and will be dependent on whether the child is entitled to support from social services. This is the English definition of 'carer':

> The word 'carer' refers to people who provide unpaid care to a relative, friend or neighbour who is in need of support because of mental or physical illness, old age or disability. (SCIE, 2005)

Additionally, in England the 1995 Carers Act introduced the term 'regular and substantial care', stating that informal (family or friends) who provided unpaid care on this basis to any disabled person would qualify as a carer under the terms of the Act.

Every parent, naturally, provides that regular and substantial care to their child in the early stages of life, and so the care provided to a disabled child may not strike the parent as being in a different category. Thus the subjective move from being a parent to becoming a 'carer' is often not a clear-cut, definite step. Williams and Robinson (2000) carried out qualitative, grounded theory research about the impact of the 1995 Carers Act on parents of people with learning disabilities. The parents whose youngsters were still children tended not to see themselves as carers, and saw this term as implying that their child was marked out as 'different'. They wanted their child with learning disabilities to be seen as just one of the family, and so their own role was simply that of 'parent'. By contrast, many older parents of people with learning disabilities retrospectively saw their whole parental life as one of challenge and struggle, on behalf of their son or daughter with learning disabilities. These parents saw themselves as fighters, and remained amazingly active and resilient. However, this study also found that one-third of the 60 parents interviewed had their own illnesses or long-term conditions amounting to a disability, and a quarter of them were carers for more than one disabled person. It is worrying that a very similar picture was expressed by 151 carers who took part in a survey and focus groups in 2010 (Mansell *et al.*, 2010). It seems that recent carer-focused legislation is having least effect, then, among family carers of adults with learning disabilities. The lifelong nature of caring responsibilities is often described as 'from their cradle to our grave', and is possibly becoming more prominent in English social care policy, with the introduction of personal budgets and direct payments (DH, 1996; 2006). Gant (2010) found that carers over the age of 60 were still concerned about the paucity and low quality of services, and felt happier to keep their adult child at home, with a gradually developing mutual care relationship building up (Williams and Robinson, 2001b).

Studies about families of people with learning disabilities thus report a mixed picture, depending largely on the purpose and outlook of the research itself. There are plenty of interpretative studies reported above, which highlight the advocacy role played by families, and also the ways in which a disabled child can impact positively on a family. However, other research has consistently shown how stressful it can be to bring up a child with learning disabilities, and indeed to support them further in adulthood. The 151 parents who reported their concerns in Mansell *et al.* (2010) had worries about information and services, suitable provision at school level, but overwhelmingly they had worries about the future and what would happen when the family was no longer able to support their relative with learning disabilities. Hill and Rose (2009) followed a more direct approach, in measuring the stress levels of 44 mothers of adults with learning disabilities, and found considerable variations in parenting stress, which could be mediated both by the parents' ability to find their own solutions, and also by service supports. It may well be that parents can report positively on their own ability to find solutions, while at the same time experiencing extreme negative consequences of their caring role. For instance, in a large Australian study, Burton-Smith (2009) found that family carers did not consider it a 'burden' to care for their relative with learning disabilities. Nevertheless, these 448 family carers had higher levels of unemployment than other groups, and lower family incomes. Their own health, and in particular their mental health, had often suffered as a result. These findings echo our own in England, some ten years previously (Williams and Robinson, 2000), and so it is fair to conclude that policy for carer support still has much to achieve at an international level.

Getting the balance right between parent and disabled person

Families in Western societies in general have an ambiguous relationship with the state. Families are private units, bringing up children who belong to them, and partaking of services such as education and health – until something goes wrong. The state considers itself, fundamentally, responsible for the welfare of all children and 'vulnerable' adults, and therefore a line can be crossed in which families cease to be seen as partners. They become, in effect, the problem, and that is when child or adult protection procedures are put into action. Recent mixed methods research by the author (Williams *et al.*, 2012) found for instance that best interests decisions under the Mental Capacity Act (see Chapter 8), were sometimes prompted by conflicts, suspicions of abuse or financial misdemeanours, by families of people with learning disabilities. Similarly, the rights of parents to act for their children are considered sacrosanct, until the rights of the child are contravened or put into jeopardy (Tarleton, 2004). As Kellett (2011: 123) points out, family problems can be flipped into 'problem families' who then are held responsible for the failures of their offspring.

The sensitivity of this situation arises from the centrality of families to the social care and support of their relative with learning disabilities. If no family members continued to 'care', then the system of social support for all disabled people would most certainly not be sufficient. However, at the same time, the state takes a primary interest in the well-being of the disabled person, and their family members are at best only seen as adjuncts. In official UK policy, for instance, the words 'and family carers' are frequently tagged on to the end of policy statements. Thus adult protection processes will focus on the welfare of the disabled person, and that can cut across, or in fact problematize, the family's input into that welfare.

In extreme cases, local authorities have such concerns about the safety and welfare of the disabled person, that safeguarding procedures are brought into play. Mansell *et al.* (2009) found that adult protection procedures identified many more cases than previously estimated. In particular, sexual abuse, though also financial, physical or psychological abuse were identified within families. Little is known about the point of view of family members who find themselves in these situations, and even less about the views of people with learning disabilities who are 'protected' from their families. However, ongoing doctoral research by a family member (Coles, ongoing) is examining the intense anger and upset that can be caused by accusations against families who have been sacrificing their very livelihoods in order to protect and manage their relative's support services.

The protection of people with learning disabilities in the past has problematized the family even more than it does now. Walmsley and Rolph (2001) show from historical records and accounts that the basis of that relationship during the twentieth century was often one of suspicion and castigation. Parents were held responsible for their children's 'faults', and moreover, they were frequently assessed, observed, and judged by public bodies to ensure that they were fit to care for their own children. While we might hope that such attitudes are a thing of the past, it is interesting to note how often parents talk of their feelings of guilt and blame, as if their child's impairment is used to throw doubt on their own integrity or skill as parents:

> Against every standard, every situation, the 'mom' gets evaluated right along with her son. Implied diagnoses of 'lazy', 'disorganized', 'failure', 'ignorant' etc. leave their scars too. (Foster-Gallasso, 2005: 22)

There are similarities in families' experiences in other countries, despite many important differences in societal attitudes, legislation and provision for disabled children. Kaplan (2010) for instance, documents that as recently as 2002, parents of children born with impairments in Russia were encouraged to leave them in state-run orphanages (Kaplan, 2010: 716). The stress on Russian families (and particularly mothers) of bringing up a disabled child is compounded by negativity in society's attitudes and total uncertainty about the future, lack of adult services, and isolation. However, as in other countries, including Australia (Plant and Sanders, 2007), China (Mak and Ho, 2007) and Canada (King *et al.*, 1999), Kaplan found that social and emotional support for mothers of disabled children was the key to enabling them to cope.

Despite the calls for partnership and family support, then, there is a point at which the needs and best interests of the person with learning disabilities take precedence over the needs of the family. Abuse, conflicts of interest, and sheer lack of ability to bring up a child with learning disabilities can still be problems in some cases, and so child and adult protection services have a huge responsibility in both supporting the family, but also safeguarding the best interests and rights of the person with learning disabilities. There is, however, very little evidence about how these procedures impact directly on families (Mansell *et al.*, 2009) or on the people with learning disabilities at the heart of these disputes (Williams *et al.*,

2012). The following section will explore in general some of the ways in which partnership work can be fostered, while keeping the needs and best interests of the person with learning disabilities at the 'centre' of that partnership.

Partnership in practice

Partnership in the early years and childhood

Parents of children with learning disabilities are recruited early on as 'partners', in their own children's socialization, development and education. Some, too, have vital roles in maintaining their children's health and well-being, particularly those whose children have profound and multiple dependencies. However, families have often found a 'whole family approach' sadly lacking (Townsley *et al.*, 2004).

What, then, does good 'partnership working' look like in the early years? It is now recognized that partnership with families is primarily about a coordinated approach, with a central key worker providing the link with the myriad of other services that might be offered to a youngster with learning disabilities. The 'Early Support' programme (DCSF, 2007c) includes several features that are worth noting:

1. A commitment to provide training in coordinated multi-agency working, which includes family members and professionals learning alongside each other.
2. A family fact-file, where families can take control of the situation by recording their own views, details of their child, and preferences. This means that they do not have to repeat everything to each new professional.
3. On-line materials and resources available to families and to professionals alike.
4. Parent workshops and information sharing, which are intended to treat parents as expert partners. The principles of 'Early Support' are outlined in Box 5.3.

Early Support training programmes are offered jointly, to professionals and parents working together, and cover the principles and values underpinning support services, legislation and policy, and the practices of partnership working.

Box 5.3	The principles of the 'Early Support' programme (2007) Partnership with parents

1. Working closely together, with active participation and involvement
2. Sharing power, with parents leading
3. Complementary expertise
4. Negotiating and agreeing aims and process
5. Mutual trust and respect.

Source: www.earlysupport.org.uk

Therefore, although there is also a focus on child development, the joint responsibility and equality of the professional–parent relationship is built into the structure of the programme.

As Lacey (2001: 136) also states, in order to build an equal partnership, it may also be necessary to redress the imbalance in the power exerted by professionals and parents. In English policy, that notion of equal power has been termed 'co-production', where solutions are created directly by disabled people or their allies and families (Hunter and Ritchie, 2007). Increasingly, parents themselves are taking active roles in research and as authors, to express their own point of view. Murray (2000) for instance, writes from the perspective of a parent. She argues that educational and other services tend to see the 'problem' of disability as an individual failure. By contrast, embracing a rights-based approach to disability as a social issue will mean that professionals and parents can meet on a more equal footing. Further, Murray argues for the child's rights and perspectives to remain absolutely at the centre of this partnership.

Similarly, parents of adults with learning disabilities in Ireland were recruited as co-researchers (Walmsley et al., 2009), in order to create their own evidence base for improved dialogue with service providers, and parents such as Dawkins (2009) and Tomlinson (2012) regularly have a voice in policy and in research forums. The more 'collaborative' relationship envisaged by Langan (2011) may be about parents and families building up their own collective voice, through groups and organizations, and through peer support. However, for power to be more equally distributed, it will also be necessary for professionals to step down from their own 'expert' platform at times. In education, that can mean teachers recognizing that parents often have the correct solution to their child's needs. Parents' forums within school can help schools to change systemically for inclusion, and teacher–parent communication should be two-way. These can be genuine 'person-centred' or student-centred partnerships, in which families and professionals are working together, both with the interests of the young person with learning disabilities at heart. The ethos and tools of person-centred planning (see Chapter 7) are invaluable here, and those interested can follow up the resources listed at the end of this chapter and Chapter 7.

Parents supporting direct payments

As emphasized throughout this chapter, the role of the family of a person with learning disabilities does not cease when they reach adulthood. That role will vary according both to the particular family and the route which the person with learning disabilities themselves follows. However, when their son or daughter continues to live in the family home, the work carried out by parents of people with learning disabilities can amount to a full-scale professional job (Shearn and Todd, 1997). Those parents have to learn to be bookkeepers, administrative assistants, managers of services, as well as parents (Grant et al., 2010: 349).

The work taken on by families has increased since the 1990s in the UK. With the new policies of personalization and direct payments (see Chapter 2, pp. 21–2), many parents in the UK are moving into key roles in supporting, and maybe even managing, their son or daughter's direct payments. In new direct payments guidance (DH, 2009b), it is acknowledged that people who may lack capacity to consent can still benefit from a direct payment. In those cases, a 'suitable person' can take on this role, and in fact receive the direct payment on their behalf. That suitable person is often the parent, or another close relative. In many respects, parents in England are often keen to take back the responsibility from local councils, and arrange for themselves the services that their son or daughter may need. A moving example is given by Caroline Tomlinson, the parent of a young man with complex needs, who writes about the 'Partners in Policymaking' courses, which as she says 'have offered individuals and families an excellent lesson in helping themselves' (Tomlinson, 2012: 28).

 Voice of Experience

Joe's story: love is simply not enough

- Following a 'Partners' course, Caroline created a circle of support, inviting people in to her son Joe's life when he was just a child.
- Later on, Caroline had the support of a professional facilitator to help with Joe's circle, and, as she says: 'Joe was fortunate to be one of the first people in the country to self-direct his own support. He now has a great team of people supporting him, his own home, his own business, his own car and a great life.'
- She then describes how essential it was for everyone to know Joe's needs, to understand who he was, and to do this in a person-centred way. She found out about a group called 'PLAN' in Canada, and developed the same concept in the UK through a group called 'Our Futures'.
- Families have supported each other to start up circles for their disabled relative, and to encourage others to develop structures so that family-led support will become more sustainable.

Source: Tomlinson, 2012

More real-life examples of personalized services for people with PMLD are shown in DVD clips which are available to view on the website for Jim Mansell's report (Mansell, 2010).

The notion of 'partnership' thus rises to new levels with these families and the tasks parents take on are not inconsiderable. Many parents for instance help their son or daughter decide what supports they need, work out how the money will be spent on those supports, identify support workers and/or day activities, manage and monitor the direct payment. It is not all parents who will wish to take on this level of responsibility, and indeed, it is not all parents who can. Moreover, there is a high chance of stress associated with the massive amount of responsibility and work these tasks can entail (Coles, ongoing). Partnerships can never be equal while professionals control the rules of the system. Nevertheless, good partnership working recognizes the ongoing needs for support of all these families, with joint working which is on the family's own terms. It is hard to get this balance correct, and in England many local councils are struggling to find ways to ensure that families managing direct payments and personal budgets have the relationship they deserve with the local authority. Qualitative research for the Office for Disability Issues (Williams and Porter, 2011) found that disabled people's own organizations could provide sensitive, facilitative support not only for disabled service users, but also for families. Forty of the 80 personal budget users who took part in that study had family carers who managed their support package. Parents themselves are often the best people to share their expertise with others embarking on personal budgets, and both user-led and other voluntary organizations can enable parents to take on this role. For partnership to become a reality, however, there have to be shifts of practice on both sides of the statutory and voluntary fence. Statutory authorities have to learn how to relinquish control, in order for families to have the freedom to develop their own solutions within a joint framework. Moreover, that partnership will work out differently for each family and each circumstance. Sensitive though it may be to get it right, it is that respect for the individuality of families which will enable people with learning disabilities to have safe, personalized and individual services to support their adult lives.

Conclusion: what has 'partnership' with families achieved?

Many families of people with learning disabilities take on vital roles, as seen in this chapter, both in direct support and care of their relative, but also in fighting for the rights of the person with learning disabilities. As one parent in Williams and Robinson (2000) put it, 'If the services were right for Jenny, I would have no needs.' For social care and health services to function, parents and other family members are an indispensable part of the picture. However, families are all different, and not all have the resources, skills or will to take up these roles; in fact, the rights of the person with learning disabilities take precedence in some cases over the rights of their family. The research summarized in this chapter is largely based on accounts given by family members themselves, and reveals that their experiences and situations have not vastly changed over the past twelve years. If anything, there are indications that the involvement of some families has increased, with the personalization of services for adults with learning disabilities.

The key concept of 'partnership' is therefore a vital goal for policy, but a very tricky one to enact in practice. Like many of the terms in this book, it is far easier to talk about than to achieve. Partnership implies first an equal balance of power between at least two parties, and qualitative research has shown how difficult that is to achieve. Family members themselves often feel that they are asked to be partners, but on the terms of the local authority or the school. This is not a level playing field, since the family's life is so deeply involved with that of their relative with learning disabilities. Professionals, by contrast, can walk away. Therefore equality requires a shift in thinking, as well as a shift in power, so that parents are actually valued and respected for their expertise.

That is perhaps why the more progressive and hopeful signs of partnership development are seen within parents' own organizations, peer support groups and collective movements of families. For instance, the development of parents' rights to take part in research, or to lead their own research, gives a new voice of authority to parents. Ongoing research about support planning in England (Williams and Porter, ongoing), is finding through interviews and observations that parents and families are supporting others, through voluntary sector organizations, enabling groups and individual peer support to develop. However, there is still a lack of research to underpin the development of partnership work with families. The theoretical knowledge about partnership working in professional practice is seldom applied systematically to joint work with families. Instead, there is much sensitivity and worry about the dual role of families, first in representing people with learning disabilities directly, and, second, in providing services and supports alongside professionals. Therefore, further development and action research is needed in this field.

People with learning disabilities who speak up for their rights do not necessarily want parents and carers to dominate their own voice. Nevertheless, the joint concerns and campaigns of people with learning disabilities and family carers have brought advocacy organizations and family-led groups together in recent years in the UK. Parents who have involvement with a person-centred planning approach have testified to its value in moving forward what is important for their own young person with learning disabilities (Tomlinson, 2012; Sanderson, 2000; Chapter 7 of this book). At an individual level, partnerships with families therefore need to keep at their heart the voice, needs and personality of the individual person with learning disabilities. Understanding each individual's and their family's strengths and needs should be the main drivers for developing a partnership approach.

Reflection exercises

1. In order to discuss the issues in this chapter, it would be useful to consider the threats to partnership policies, as well as possible solutions, at the following changing points in a family's life cycle. Specifically, families are faced with very significant changes in their legal rights and their access to services at:

   - The stage of 'transition' when the child is 14–19 (see Chapter 7) when planning should start for the post-school period.
   - The age of 18, when the child officially becomes an adult, and the shift has to be made from children's services to adult services.
   - The point at which their son or daughter might move out of the family home, if that does occur (see Chapter 8). The official status of the parent generally then ceases to be that of 'carer'.
   - Changes in their own status or lifestyle. For instance, on receipt of a state pension, a carer can no longer receive a carer's allowance, but becomes officially an 'older person'.

2. A partnership approach that is truly person-centred will keep the changing needs and views of the person with learning disabilities at the foreground. As life moves on, that person will develop relationships outside the family, and the relationship within the family may change. Link this chapter with Chapter 7, to think about how person-centred approaches can help families and their relative with learning disabilities.

3. Adults with learning disabilities frequently continue to have support from parents or other family members. If you are a practitioner, consider how you yourself would work in partnership with older family carers and with other professionals. Consider particularly how carers' rights should be protected by the legislation listed in Box 5.1, and how this would affect partnership work.

Suggested further resources

1. For information and advice about families' involvement in person-centred approaches, see: www.familiesleadingplanning.co.uk/Documents/PCAFamilies.pdf

2. 'Partners in Policymaking' courses can be traced through from their USA origins at www.partnersinpolicymaking.com, and the English courses, guidance and discussion can be accessed through: www.in-control.org.uk/what-we-do/partners-in-policymaking.aspx

3. Families' own stories are very valuable, and a great collection can be found in Murray, P. and Penman, J. (eds) (2000) *Telling Our Own Stories: Reflections on Family Life in a Disabling World*, Sheffield: Parents with Attitude.

4. The Social Care Institute for Excellence (SCIE) has a section on its website for and about carers. It includes good, up-to-date information, as well as videos about family life: www.scie.org.uk/topic/careservices/carerssupport

6 Identity, Relationships, Sexuality and Parenting

'No man is an island' wrote John Donne and while we would now want to include women as well as well as men in this quote, it still holds true for most of us. The idea of isolation, of not being loved or being able to give love to others, is a frightening thought. Relationships affect how people think about themselves, and how they are seen by others. That is why the theme of identity is coupled here with an exploration of relationships.

Key points summary:

- The need to love and be loved is central in everyone's lives, and people with learning disabilities are no different.
- Other people sometimes do not think that people with learning disabilities can have feelings, nor that they can enjoy sex.
- Everyone has different relationships throughout their life.
- When people with learning disabilities take up new roles, for instance as parents, then people see them in a new light.
- That is why it is important to think about 'identities', so that people can get better support that allows them to take up new roles.

Voice of Experience

There's nobody quite like me (by Kerrie Ford)

When I was a child I got sent to special schools, because I had severe physical disabilities. And they said it was to do with memory and direction, but I didn't think I was that severely disabled. It was only when I went to college that they started using words like 'learning difficulty', and I transferred from one college to another – I've been to so many colleges. I've always felt there's nobody quite like me. I went to three different special schools, and liked to talk to the staff. I felt lonely with the people around me. Every time I wanted friends, they didn't have the same disability as me, and they seemed to think that I was different.

Relationships are the most important thing in my life. A friend is someone you can go out with, and have a laugh with. They help you with the hard things in life. I can help my friend do stuff, but sometimes it's very difficult to help.

Relationships can be controlling. For instance, I had a boyfriend who wanted to de-pick my brain, and he wanted to try and sort my brain out. He thought that counselling would help me, and his way of doing it, was to just leave it when he'd had enough. So it was a way to try and hurt me. But now I've got a friend who is quite happy with the way I am, and even though we're not boyfriend and girlfriend, we are quite close friends. And it's much better that way.

Family relationships

When I was a child, I had a relationship with my dad where he would control me. Relationships now can also be very controlling, but the best sort of relationship is when someone says: 'You don't have to revolve your life around me', and they say I can have my life as I want it. I can lead my own life, and we can meet twice a week. So that we're not in each other's pockets all the time.

My mum always stood up for me, when she could. My mum always said, that I should not have been put into a special school, I should have gone to a mainstream school where you've got ordinary people too.

That's not a control, but just a way to help me. So some control can be helpful, and some can't. It all depends on how you look at it.

Getting support with mental health

When my grandma died, my whole world fell apart. I felt as if I'd lost my trust in people. And nobody has actually gone into my brain, to see why these panic attacks started. Nobody wants to go right inside my brain, to make me feel happier and better again. I don't get that sort of support.

Support staff relationships

Back twenty years ago, support workers weren't always very good. We had support workers at school, but they weren't very good back in those days. They wanted their fag and cup of coffee, before they could function. I would tell them off for doing that, but with the disabled community, it seemed like the carers could only support them for a couple of hours before they got fed up with them.

Now things are better with support staff. My support worker tries to be like a friend, although it's not really an equal. She said to me that I should think for myself, and not just do my hair the way my mum likes it. I agree that I should make my own choices, but I also try to make my mum pleased as well.

There was one time when I went to the pictures to see *Walk the Line*, with two helpers who were friends and colleagues, and my disabled friend. I put the flags out – to say, I don't need to be supporting anyone, I can be a child. I can go and watch a film and relax. It was a good film! That's what I want in a friend, I just want to go out and do things.

Introduction and overview

Enduring personal relationships are of vital importance to all of us. They are at the centre of our emotional stability and our sense of identity. In other words they are fundamental to both the way we see ourselves and how we are seen, as Kerrie Ford explains above. She says that she felt lonely in college, as others saw her as different. This chapter is entitled Identity, Relationships, Sexuality and Parenting because these three areas of life are central and provide challenges to us all, but particularly to people with learning disabilities. Early relationships focus on our families of origin and then as we grow, include friendships with peers. Later in adolescence and adulthood we add intimate adult relationships that may be short or long term to our earlier friends and family. Then many of us add a new form of relationship in becoming parents. Integral to many of these relationships is sexuality and its expression. Accounts by people with learning disabilities about their lives reveal some of the difficulties they face in forming and developing relationships and having good and safe sexual lives. These difficulties include other people who control them, isolation from mainstream society, and people who abuse trust.

This chapter provides a particular space in the book where the voices of people with learning disabilities can be heard in narrative research about their experiences of relationships. It aims to describe the dreams and hopes some people with learning disabilities have, identify the barriers they confront in forming and sustaining meaningful relationships and to suggest some of the ways to support their dreams and hopes.

Key policy concept: identity

Theories of identity

Identity is a frequently used term, both in academic debate and at the level of personal, everyday language about human experience. However, like many of the other key terms in this book, it is slippery and can be approached in many different ways. For instance, social identity theories (Tajfel *et al.*, 1971), based on experimental methods, have shown how human beings have a tendency to *identify* with dominant social groups, and how group membership can subsequently affect the way people think about themselves. As Kerrie commented in the opening story in this chapter, she was seen as different from others in school, and so felt she was the odd one out. Whole categories of people, including disabled people, were classified in the Second World War as 'other' and were frequently denied the right to life. Therefore, identity theories are not just an academic luxury. They are essential to understanding and improving the way social and political life is conducted.

In postmodern societies, it is often assumed that identity has become fragmented and that it is socially constructed, both by the individual but also through their interaction with the way in which others view them (De Fina *et al.*, 2006: 1–23). While previously nationality, race, geographical location, family role and employment status were all key features in defining who we were, all of these features have become mixed and tend to shift over the life-course (Clarke *et al.*, 2007). Identity can be studied, then, simply by asking people about how they identify themselves. When that was attempted with people with a learning disability, however, Davies and Jenkins (1997) found that the label 'learning disability' was not generally a term people used about themselves. Rapley *et al.* (1998) subsequently commented that 'learning disability' is often used as a term of abuse, and a denial of being learning disabled does not necessarily mean that people are unaware of the label assigned to them. At the very least, this body of research about self-identification reveals how problematic the label of 'learning disability' can be for those to whom we apply it.

In discussing 'identity', there is a need to distinguish between inner cognition or consciousness of self, and the social roles that are occupied by individuals. Kerrie says 'there's nobody quite like me', and perhaps we all think of ourselves as unique. However, everyone occupies multiple roles, and will find that different aspects of their identity are salient in different circumstances. However, the experience of people with learning disabilities is not always so flexible. As Gillman *et al.* (2000) cogently argue, the diagnosis of 'learning disability' defines the individual in an all-encompassing way, overshadowing or masking the possibility of an individual occupying other roles. In this chapter, that dominant and stigmatizing aspect of a learning disability identity is very relevant, for instance in considering if and how people with learning disabilities can be considered as sexual individuals, partners or as parents.

Identity can also be studied through human communication. Some branches of discourse analysis (Potter, 2003; Wetherell, 1998) examine the fine-grained detail of interactions in social settings, to show how categories of identity can shift on a moment-by-moment basis in the fluid course of a conversation (Antaki and Widdicombe, 1998). For instance, in marriage guidance counselling, Greatbatch and Dingwall (1998) show how each partner makes relevant their own and each other's identities, using these frameworks in some respects to present their case. Each encounter both builds on, and re-colours, the way in which each person thinks about themselves, how they 'invoke or accept or contest the relevance of identities on a moment to moment basis' (Greatbatch *et al.*, 1998:131).

Kerrie, at the end of her story at the top of this chapter, clearly valued going out with friends, so that she could 'relax'. For a person with learning disabilities, then, each new encounter and each new relationship will offer them a fresh chance to define themselves, as it does for everyone. In Williams (2011) evidence for that position is explored in greater depth. For now, however, it should be noted that the identity of 'learning disability' can both dominate and restrict people with that label. In order to understand that position, the central arguments about identity in disability studies generally will be outlined next.

Identity and disability

Concepts of identity are at the heart of disability theory, which has reframed and critiqued the way 'disability' in general is constructed by society (Barnes and

Mercer, 2006: 2–4). The argument of social model theorists (see Chapter 2) challenges previous views of what it meant to be disabled, where the problem was situated within the person. A disabled identity, in the medical 'model', is a deficient, problematic identity (Oliver, 1990). Arguing for a reframing of disability as a social problem, these theorists have thus addressed identity as a social issue, challenging the fact that disabled people are collectively positioned in certain ways by others in society. Demanding the right to define one's own identity is both a challenge but an essential part of any collective movement for change. Interestingly, social movements have often used a previously devalued label, such as 'queer' or 'black' to define their identity, and it essentially becomes a badge of pride.

However, with some exceptions, people with learning disabilities have had some difficulty in establishing pride in their identity. As Chappell (2000) argues, they were not originally included within the social model, nor within the disabled people's movement (Walmsley, 1997). Nevertheless, the self-advocacy movement (see Chapter 2) has provided a vehicle for their own collective voice, and indeed labelling and identity issues have from the start been a central focus of that movement. People with learning disabilities face challenges and barriers stemming both from their own impairment, and from the ways in which society favours intellectual ability. The result is often that they are treated in ways that do not allow them to identify entirely with other disabled people who do not have cognitive impairments.

In England and other Western societies in the twenty-first century, people with learning disabilities are therefore still regularly treated as less than full members of society. Despite the demands of people with learning disabilities to be seen as 'people first', through their own collective self-advocacy movement, society's view of what it means to have a learning disability impinges on their experience on a day-to-day basis, in encounters with staff (see Chapter 9 of this book; Williams, 2011; Rapley 2004; Antaki et al., 2007b) and within policy debates about learning disability. For instance, the identity of 'learning disability' and the very definition in UK government policy (see p. 15) is premised on the notion that people are incapable and need a degree of support and protection to manage everyday life. There are no easy answers here, since the needs arising from the impairment of 'learning disability' have to be considered alongside arguments about social barriers and rights. Nevertheless, by supporting people with learning disabilities to take up diverse roles, through relationships, friendships and employment, people with the label of 'learning disability' can gradually view themselves in new ways and challenge the view that society holds about them.

Relationships and identity therefore are closely interlinked, and lie at the heart of developing policy and practice with people with learning disabilities. It will be argued later in this chapter that identity considerations are central in effective support for the social and relational aspects of people's lives. First, though, the following section will review some of the body of evidence about how people with learning disabilities experience relationships and sexuality in their lives, and in doing so, will highlight the direct voices of individuals with learning disabilities themselves.

Research evidence about relationships for people with learning disabilities

Family relationships

For most of us our family of origin (parents, siblings and other extended family members) is an important part of our lives, often for extended periods that go well beyond childhood, and even when we leave home to take up work or to develop long-term adult relationships. Our relationships with members of our family of origin change over time. For example as we enter middle life we may find ourselves in a role reversal situation where we become the carers for older family members.

However, adult relationships with their family of origin may be different for people with learning disabilities. For example, as seen in Chapter 5, around half of adults with learning disabilities continue to live with parents, well into their own adulthood and into their parents' old age (Gant, 2010).

A close relationship with parents and other family members is something that is often assumed and naturalized into the way people with learning disabilities live. It is often a relationship based on long-term dependency, and one that may be close – but can also be difficult at times for both parties, as Kerrie Ford points out in the opening story in this chapter. Marie Wolfe, a woman with learning disabilities living in Ireland, also wrote about the importance of parents stepping back and allowing their son or daughter to get on with their own life:

 Voice of Experience

I have a good relationship with my parents … They even said to me once: 'you might get married'. It [surprised me] like. As long as I seem to be getting on well, they keep out of it. They don't really talk to any staff or anything, they don't interfere or anything. It's good, like. Not many parents are like that, you know.

Source: Wolfe, in Johnson *et al.*, 2010: 19

As was explored in Chapter 5, parents and other family members are often central to the life chances of their son or daughter with learning disabilities, in the UK and in other countries. However, that relationship has some significant features, which are a result of the roles that parents have to play throughout their child's life, and into adulthood. These include a strong emphasis on 'caring', including physical care, a continued role as educator, spanning many aspects of life and independence skills, advocacy in fighting for rights and services, and protection from risk. From the point of view of the adult with learning disabilities, it is therefore very hard to conceive of a parent who steps down from these roles and both encourages and supports their sexual relationships. That is why Marie Wolfe was surprised, in the quotation above, by her parents' comment about marriage.

Taking part in decisions as to how adult people with learning disabilities will live in the community and being involved in an ongoing way with the services they use can add to already complex and difficult relationships. Parents in Williams, Simons *et al.* (2005) whose son or daughter had a personal assistant and was living independently, said that they felt relieved that they could at last simply 'be parents', rather than having to be a service provider and supporter. However, very little is known about how that relationship between adults and parents is experienced by the person with learning disabilities. As Kerrie Ford mentioned in her account, her relationship with her parents continues to play an important role in her life even though she has moved out of the parental home, and that was also so for Anya Souza (1997; and see Chapter 5, pp. 82–4). With some increased distance, it can be easier for both parties to 'let go' and enjoy their relationship.

One of the fears of older parents with an adult son or daughter with learning disabilities is the anxiety about what will become of them when their parents die. However, Bigby (1997, 2000) found that for some older women life became more varied and open once they had left the care of their parents. So Vera began a new life after her parents' death:

> Vera has become more independent. She just does things that she would never have dreamt of doing once upon a time. [sister of Vera aged 69 who lives in an 'aged' person's hostel] (Bigby, 2000: 71)

As seen in Chapter 5, siblings also play an important role in people's lives, and that ongoing relationship with a brother or sister can be vital to people with learning disabilities, whatever their living situation, often leading to new roles as aunt or uncle to their siblings' families.

People with learning disabilities as carers

Perhaps one of the least acknowledged relationships between people with learning disabilities and their families is the caring role that some people with learning disabilities play in relation to their older parents or with a partner. There is a tendency to see people with learning disabilities as being cared for rather than as being carers

Voice of Experience

Ooh, me dad died five years afore. It was after me dad died me mum got rheumatoid arthritis. I had to do housework, cooking, she couldn't get out see, we lived on a hill, top of a hill, she got rheumatoid arthritis in her knees ... except when me brother fetched her, fetched her in the car she never got out ... I mean she was 'ousebound ... my mum was very ill, cancer ... I knew it were coming.

Source: 'Beryl', in Walmsley, 2000: 202

themselves. Yet there is evidence from people with learning disabilities themselves and from family members that some people become carers for their ageing parents or are involved in mutual caring relationships with a partner (Bigby, 2000; Walmsley, 1993; Williams and Robinson, 2001b). One woman with learning disabilities describes her care of her older mother at the bottom of page 98.

While Beryl seems to have been supported in her caring role by other family members, necessitating in some way a division of roles and a partnership to ensure that her mother was supported, some people with learning disabilities have been left to take sole responsibility for arranging care for older parents. Colin, who had no family other than his mother, became responsible for her support, at first as she lived alone in her own home, then in hospital and finally in the search for a nursing home. Without support from a personal friend Colin would have found the situation impossible. He says:

It is to be hoped that a best interests decision made for Colin's mother would now

Voice of Experience

When we saw the social worker, they were trying to get mum out of hospital within 24 hours. We just couldn't do that. That's when I think, I asked Rosy, you know: 'What the hell am I going to do?' John next door told us about the place at Bell Haven [a nursing home for older people]. So Rosy and I went up and had a look and there was a place. Rosy checked out a couple of other places. I couldn't go with her. She did that as my friend, a really good friend.

Source: Hiscoe with Johnson, 2007: 167

take into account Colin's own views and his needs (see Chapter 8). In his life story Colin stresses the need for partnership support with professional workers which would have made his experience with his mother less stressful, allowed Rosy not to take on a caring role and would have given him more time to be a son with his mother.

Friendships

Voice of Experience

I think one thing I'm missing here is friendship. Either male or female it doesn't matter. Either a male or female friend, I don't mind. I prefer something like companionship.

Source: David Warren, in Johnson *et al.*, 2001: 70

David lived with minimal support independently in the community, but although he had a job he found that people never contacted him, never dropped in or suggested going out. In social situations he found it difficult to maintain a conversation and found that he was quickly isolated at the pub or at other social events. David is not alone in his longing for companionship and friendship and in his loneliness.

In exploring how people with learning disabilities experience friendship, and the barriers they may face, it is important to have some sense of the nature of friendship. While we all recognize a friend, it can be quite difficult to identify what characterizes this relationship. The number and type of friendships that we develop over time varies with the individual. For some people it is important to have a close relationship with just a few people, but for others a wide circle of friends is important.

Both acquaintances and friends serve a number of different purposes in our lives:

- Company
- Opportunities for experience
- A sense of self identity
- Self esteem
- Practical help

(Firth and Rapley, 1990: 18)

Firth and Rapley go on to identify five characteristics that they believe are important in defining friends as opposed to acquaintances:

1. **Choice.** We do not choose our family members and often we do not choose our acquaintances either, but we do tend to choose those whom we regard as friends.
2. **Mutuality.** There is an equality or reciprocity in friendship. In some relationships positive feelings may be held by one party and not by the other. This cannot be said about friendship.
3. **Commitment**. Friends spend time together out of choice, share joys and sorrows and are willing to give their relationship an important priority.
4. **Persistence**. Friendship is ongoing, continuing over a longer period of time than that of acquaintances or indeed some intimate sexual relationships.
5. **Intimacy**. Shared values and a willingness to give of oneself are important in the development of friendship.

Similarly Kerrie in her opening story, comments on the mutuality and reciprocity involved in friendship: 'A friend is someone you can go out with, and have a laugh with. They help you with the hard things in life.'

Adults often form friendships through social events or through work. This is also true for people with learning disabilities. For example Janice, in Slattery with Johnson (2000), met her friend Amanda as a result of them both working for advocacy organizations. However many people with learning disabilities do not have the same work opportunities for friendships to develop (Jenner and Gale,

2006). Partly as a result of this they tend to have much smaller social networks than others in the community, as quantitative research (Emerson *et al.*, 2005; Robertson *et al.*, 2001a) and in-depth ethnographic research (Pockney, 2006) have shown. Such networks have, in some research, been found to be less long term than those of others in the community and are mainly made up of staff, families and other people with learning disabilities (Forrester-Jones *et al.*, 2006). It is therefore hardly surprising that people with learning disabilities often count their staff members as friends (Pockney, 2006; Antaki *et al.*, 2007b). Few of the staff in Pockney (2006) reciprocated this attribution when describing the people with learning disabilities with whom they worked, although other research has examined how relationships between people with learning disabilities and their personal assistants can take place on a basis of equality and indeed friendliness (Ponting *et al.*, 2010; see also Chapter 9). The blurred boundary between friendship and professional support can be confusing, but those in Ponting *et al.* (2010) agree with Felt, below, that *some* relationships with staff members can become friendships:

> All in all I do know that there are some assistants who are my friends. They may say or do things I don't like sometimes, but I do know they're my friends. They've stuck by me for a long time. (Felt with Walker, 2000: 223)

Barriers to friendship

The barriers that people with learning disabilities may encounter in developing friendships as adults have been identified in research as both social and as being particular characteristics of the individual, thus drawing both on a social model and an individual model of disability (see Chapter 2). A statistical analysis of over 1,500 adults living in supported accommodation suggests that the place in which someone lives may be a stronger factor in determining the quality and the extent of friendship networks than an individual's characteristics (Emerson & McVilly, 2005). The segregation involved in institutional life made it impossible for many people with learning disabilities to find friendships outside their immediate day to day living environment, although people did form close relationships with some of those with whom they lived (Johnson, 1998). One of the hopes of the deinstitutionalization movement was that people would form more relationships once they were living in the community. However this does not always happen. A longitudinal study of people who had moved from institutions into the community found that this movement did not generally result in social inclusion (Forrester-Jones *et al.*, 2006), although those living in smaller, community based settings had larger and more inclusive social networks in a sample of 500 adults (Robertson *et al.*, 2001a).

Attitudes of other community members are also important. David Warren (p. 99 above), found it difficult to sustain relationships within the community in part because of the attitudes of those around him. Other people with learning disabilities have also written of the difficulties they encounter from others with whom they may hope to make friends. Daniel Docherty writes of his experiences as an adult in relation to friendships and concludes that he is now wary of being with people who do not have learning disabilities.

Voice of Experience

When I became an adult I had a few non-disabled friends but some of them only spoke to me when they wanted something, like money ...

Now I've got one long term friend, he's been my friend for fifteen years; he's a disabled person. We've got a lot in common because we're both disabled. I don't seem to stay friends with non-disabled people very long, I'm always thinking what do they want, is this genuine? They buy me dinner, what do they want in return?

Source: Carson and Docherty, 2002: 144

Research has also underlined the lack of opportunity that people with learning disabilities have to meet others and develop friendships, as outlined in Box 6.1. These figures suggest a group of people who do not have access to many of the environments in which friends are commonly made.

Box 6.1   Living and employment situations of people with learning disabilities

- About half of adults with learning disabilities live with their families of origin (Chapter 5, in this book).
- In 2005, about one in three people with learning disabilities were living in some form of supported accommodation, and of those, 62 per cent were in residential care homes, and a small proportion (3 per cent) still in hospitals.
- About 11,000 of these people live out of area, that is away from their home area (Chapter 8, in this book).
- Seventeen per cent of people with learning disabilities who are of working age have a paid job.

Source: Emerson *et al.*, 2005; see Chapter 10 in this book

People with learning disabilities living in private households are likely to live in areas characterized by high levels of social deprivation. Particularly those with mild or moderate learning disabilities, living independently, experience higher than average financial hardship as compelling research with over 10,000 British young people has shown (Emerson and Hatton, 2007b). Living in areas of social deprivation, and with the majority of people with learning disabilities dependent on disability pensions and benefits, means that opportunities for taking advantage of social opportunities can be limited because of financial constraints. However, Tilly (2011) is exploring with a group of people with learning disabilities their ability to cope with everyday life on reduced incomes, and has found that friendship and peer support are vital elements for them.

Research also suggests that there are individual characteristics that may make it difficult for some people with learning disabilities to develop adult friendships. Among the characteristics of individuals that have been identified as having an impact on friendships and social networks are:

- *The age of the person.* Younger people have tended to have larger social networks than older people (Robertson *et al.*, 2001; Abraham, *et al.*, 2002). Robertson *et al.'s* multivariate analysis suggested that for younger people in particular, while family support for community participation was beneficial in developing social networks, going out as a family member did not assist this development. These findings also suggested the need for support for older adults to develop social networks.
- *Impairment-related issues.* People with autism have been found to have smaller social networks than other people (Robertson *et al.*, 2001; Knott *et al.*, 2006). Those who have higher abilities are more likely to have diverse social networks (Robertson *et al.*, 2001; Hall *et al.*, 2005). Finally those people who show 'challenging behaviour' may find it more difficult to be socially included than those who do not (Robertson *et al.*, 2001).

Sexuality and intimate relationships

 Voices of Experience

I got married in St Leos. Our anniversary is coming up soon in April. Five years now. It was a happy day. I was very happy. I like being married. Rob's got some disabilities. We were at special school together. We help each other, shopping and things like that, budgeting. Budgeting and that stuff. Sometimes we do things together, sometimes not. Sometimes we fight, but not real fighting ... But we get together again. Sometimes we argue ... I think every couple argues sometimes. It's not normal if you don't.
Source: Alicia Rodriguez, in Johnson *et al.*, 2001: 75

Oh I miss her. Oh I really miss her, oh I know I can cook, but I know I can cook, but I really miss her cookin'. Oh bein' with her and watchin' TV and stuff like that. Oh goin' shoppin' with her. Goin' for a drive with her mum, stuff like that. Oh we cuddle, yeah I miss that stuff too, cuddlin' and kissin'. I miss that stuff too ... I miss, miss, miss havin' sex , sex with Simone. Havin' sex and havin' fun with her.
Source: Darren Smith, in Johnson *et al.*, 2001: 70

Alicia and Darren are two people with learning disabilities who express the range of emotions that are representative of feelings about long-term or longed-for relationships. Not everyone wants such a relationship. Some people enjoy the expression of their sexuality through short-term relationships or casual encounters or by self-stimulation. However, it needs to be recognized that most people with learning disabilities as they move into adulthood will have a need for some form of sexual expression and many want a close and intimate relationship with someone else.

Although we are confronted with sexual imagery on TV and in newspapers every day, sexuality remains a difficult concept to define. While there have been debates among theorists and writers about its nature, about when it begins and how it should be expressed (for a good discussion, see McCarthy, 1999), the ways in which we express ourselves can be seen as:

- Enjoyment of touch of ourselves and others and a physical release.
- The development of intimate relationships with other(s). For some people this will be a heterosexual relationship and for others a same-sex one or both.
- Procreation or having children.

People with learning disabilities face many barriers to enjoyment of a sex life. In some Western countries (up until 1970s in Iceland) women leaving institutions were required to undergo sterilization to ensure that they did not have children (Sigurjonsdottir, 2000). Although eugenics (see Chapter 2) is now discredited as theory it does emerge through some of the attitudes that are still held about the sexuality of people with learning disabilities. This finds its outlet in views that they may be sexually promiscuous or dangerous and in a conflation of sexual expression and having children.

Living in different cultures can vary the emphasis placed on different aspects of sexuality. So procreation in some countries or groups may be seen as the main aim of sexual relationships. For other cultures and groups the pleasures of touch and physical release may be the most important aspect. Recognizing that we all have different views about sexuality is important in thinking about people with learning disabilities as the way those around them frame their own sexual values may impact on how they support or work with a person with learning disabilities. The example in Box 6.2 illustrates this.

Not many countries make such direct prohibitions about sexuality and people with learning disabilities as in Ireland. However some forms of sexual expression were, at least until recently in many countries, forbidden by law, for example same-sex relationships. Such proscriptions reveal the way in which we culturally limit what is seen as acceptable sexual behaviour. Some of these proscriptions while now not in force legally, remain issues for people with learning disabilities. For example while they may now not be legally banned, same-sex relationships remain difficult to acknowledge openly in some countries, and Abbott and Howarth (2002) found that in the UK same-sex relationships between people

| Box 6.2 | **Ireland: Sexual Offences Act 1993** |

In the Republic of Ireland the Sexual Offences Act 1993 makes it illegal to have penetrative sex with people with learning disabilities unless they are married. This law which sought to protect people from abuse or exploitation has had the effect of making it very difficult for service providers or families to support people with learning disabilities to have sexual relationships or indeed to provide them with sex education. Although no one has been charged under the Act, it has served to constrain people's sexual lives.

This Act was not designed deliberately to exclude people with learning disabilities from having sexual relationships. Rather, it was seen as a protection for them from abuse or exploitation.

with learning disabilities were often not even recognized as such by staff who supported them. Additionally, even when people with learning disabilities identified as gay or lesbian (Abbott and Howarth, 2002), they found it hard to access gay or lesbian social life. It would seem that the identity as 'learning disabled' was more important to most people they encountered than their identity as 'gay', and that it was difficult to combine the two characteristics for many people.

Proscriptions about sexuality are often driven by concerns about possible abuse. Research has revealed that people with learning disabilities are more likely to be exploited or abused sexually than other citizens (McCarthy, 1999). Most often such abuse or exploitation is by someone known to the person. In countries where such abuse has been discovered it can lead to increased supervision and restriction of people's lives in an effort to ensure that this does not happen. For example abuse was the main reason for the passing of the Irish Act referred to above. Unfortunately the protection and the barriers to sexual expression which are then implemented can restrict people's freedom. In a climate of prohibition they may lead lives hidden from those around them and become even more vulnerable to abuse. However, gradually this situation is changing with for example accounts suggesting that current parents of teenagers are increasingly liberal and supportive in considering relationship issues for their sons and daughters (Rogers, 2010).

People with learning disabilities as parents

 Voices of Experience

It's always better towards the end [of pregnancy] because it seems real. You know that it's real. This one's different too, and when it kicks and moves I think, oh wow, it's a real baby. And you can actually kind of picture it. I can picture myself as a mother again.

Source: Merrilyn, mother with learning disabilities, cited in Maye and Sigurjonsdottir, 2010: 22

I had two children. The Welfare took them. I had one when I was 17. No, one when I was 19 ... The Welfare took them. They'll never find my kids ... Gave the first baby a hug but not the second. I miss them.

Source: Vicki Mulholland, mother with learning disabilities, cited in Johnson *et al.*, 2000b: 43

It was a joint decision [not to have kids] and that decision was made by me and my husband. I had the tubal ligation in 1983 and soon after I had that I felt this tremendous ... I still can't even describe it even today. I had a great big burden off my shoulders.

Source: Amanda Millear with Johnson, 2000: 244–5

The views about parenting held by people with learning disabilities are as diverse and passionate as those of the rest of the population. Some people, like Amanda, have actively chosen not to be parents. She was clear that she did not want to have a child. The joy of becoming a mother to a wanted child is clear in Merrilyn's statement and the sense of loss and pain at losing children is still present for Vicki even though close to twenty years have passed since her children were taken from her.

While sterilization through surgery is now either banned or heavily hedged by legalities in most countries, there are still accounts of young women who are sterilized or are coerced into having abortions (Traustadottir and Sigurjonsdottir, 2010). Further, although many people with learning disabilities live in the community, becoming a parent remains a difficult issue for people with learning disabilities. For example research has established that there are high rates (40–60 per cent) of child removal from parents with learning disabilities (Booth *et al.*, 2005; Elvish *et al.*, 2006).

In England there has been a shift in policy relating to people with learning disabilities and a recognition of their right to parent and to have support to do so. *Valuing People* states:

> People with learning disabilities can be good parents and provide their children with a good start in life but may require considerable support to do so. This requires children and adult support teams to work closely together to develop a common approach. (DH, 2001: para 7.40)

Research suggests that 'most parents with learning disabilities have mild to borderline cognitive limitations' (McConnell *et al.*, 2010: 244). They can include people who have previously lived in institutions, those who have had a lifetime of support services, but also those who have not previously used any services but who are identified as having learning disabilities on becoming parents. There is now in-depth and inclusive research evidence which supports the view that many parents with learning disabilities are capable of being 'good enough' parents, especially when provided with good ongoing emotional and practical support (McGaw and Newman, 2005). Good support practices will be explored further below. However, in spite of these findings, people with learning disabilities do face a number of challenges in taking on a parenting role.

As noted above between 40 and 60 per cent of parents with learning disabilities have their children taken from them. This perhaps reflects a perceived tension between supporting parents and protecting children. The issue is not however clear cut. While some surveys of research on parents with learning disabilities suggest that some children of parents with learning disabilities are at risk of lack of good care or are vulnerable to abuse and neglect (James, 2004), other literature surveys (Tarleton *et al.*, 2006) provide a different picture. Their review of the literature found that these perceived risks to children may not be supported by evidence.

Whatever the case, it is undoubtedly true that parents with learning disabilities frequently face threats of losing their child, and the difficulties of child protection procedures. Booth *et al.* (2005) examined court records to explore the incidence of people with learning disabilities coming before the Family Courts and the outcomes for these families. Their study revealed that parents with learning disabilities were disproportionately represented in the Family Courts with one in every six children at Family Court having at least one parent with a learning disability. However when the reasons for the court action were analysed 47 per cent of these cases were found to be due to misguided parenting rather than to actual abuse and the vast majority of cases were brought due to charges of neglect which may be related to poverty and lack of support.

Some studies have sought the views of parents with learning disabilities about the loss of their children (Booth *et al.*, 2005; Baum and Burns, 2007). The studies revealed common themes from parents.

- Lack of support in relation to parenting and in relation to court proceedings.
- Inappropriate assessments of the parents that were often written in inaccessible language and tended to focus on possible deficits.
- Lack of advocacy for parents leading to silencing of their voice in proceedings.
- Lack of clear messages from professionals. Sometimes feedback to parents was very different from the material presented in court reports.
- Lack of support to help parents if their child was taken from them.
- Lack of time given to parents in preparing for court cases or during them.

Booth *et al.* (2005) found that many professionals involved with the families focused on the parent's learning disability rather than on evidence for neglect. The court records suggested that many parents had been offered little or no support and there was a feeling from professionals that such support would not be useful. However, such a view is not supported by evidence from qualitative research that people with learning disabilities can make loving and supportive parents. It is therefore vital to find ways to work together to support relationships, sexuality and parenting, and these will be outlined in the following section.

Practice: respecting and supporting relationships

Changing social views of a 'learning disabled' identity

In order to ensure that people with learning disabilities enjoy more friendships and other social relationships, some systemic changes are needed. For instance, communities need to develop within which people with learning disabilities feel included and safe in developing friendships. That may mean developments of community links that go beyond specialized and segregated services, and ensuring that there are community spaces and activities within which people with learning disabilities can participate. For example, Coles *et al.* (2005) explored community settings in which people with learning disabilities could have meaningful activities, and these are described further in Chapter 10 of this book. In the 'Community Connecting' initiative, some individuals with the most complex needs found roles where they could contribute to their communities. In doing so, people can be supported to change the view society has of them, from one of dependent service user to an active contributor. That shift of identity promotes confidence and a new sense of self, which can then be the basis for new relationships.

Specific initiatives focused on individuals or groups can also help to address the isolation in which many people with learning disabilities find themselves. For instance, there is some evidence that some forms of social skills training may assist young people with learning disabilities. Young people in an action research study by Williams and Heslop (2006) claimed that friends were at the centre of their support networks, and that they would turn to a friend as a first port of call, to confide their troubles. A young people's research group in that study developed a short course which was delivered by other people with learning disabilities. They found that it helped young people with learning disabilities to talk more freely about feelings and build confidence and mutual trust.

Supporting individuals with learning disabilities to learn new social skills has to go hand in hand with ensuring that structures are there for them to meet new people and develop their relationships. On-line dating agencies have in general become very popular in the UK and other countries, and there is no reason why people with learning disabilities should not use them. However, concerns are often expressed about their safety, and the possibility of abuse. Therefore, specific dating agencies and friendship groups can take care to check on all customers, and ensure a safer service for people with learning disabilities. A dating agency such as Stars in the Sky (see end of this chapter) may provide opportunities for extending social networks, and perhaps developing close relationships.

All these attempts to support relationships have to be seen in the context of specific cultures. In 2004, an EU Grundtvig project reported on a two-year collaborative project to develop training materials for people with learning disabilities about relationships and sexuality (Grundtvig, 2006). Each country in that project had a different stance towards sexuality in relation to people with learning disabilities, and so the final output incorporated both the protective attitude of some countries, and the more open and facilitative attitude prevalent in other parts of Europe. The importance of considering cultural and social factors in relation to sexuality is emphasized in the following account of sexuality offered in a government policy in Australia.

> Sexuality has psychological, emotional and reproductive aspects that are influenced by gender, class, politics, religion, social and cultural factors. A person's understanding of their sexuality is central to their self image and self awareness as well as impacting greatly on how they relate to themselves and others. A person's sexual behaviour should be viewed in the context of overall personal and social development, knowledge and skills. (Strategic Planning and Development Unit Disability Services, Tasmania, 2001: 4)

Supporting people to develop new relationships

Changing attitudes towards relationship building for people with learning disabilities has to be supported in practical ways. For instance, it can be difficult for two people with learning disabilities to get to see each other in their own homes, if they are entirely dependent on transport provided by their parents or service providers. Further, some people living in 'supported living' or independent settings are offered very rigid timetables of day activities, with the hours of support they need coming in at regular times. This can make it difficult to accept an invitation from a friend, or to spontaneously go out to a social venue and meet new friends. Therefore, good practice in developing relationships is not simply about acceptance and hope that friendships will happen; it is also about providing the practical support in a way that will enable people to have the freedom for their own social life. This is a delicate balancing act for support workers who need to find ways to be supportive but at the same time step back so that the person they support has opportunities to develop friendships and relationships on their own terms (Ponting *et al.*, 2010).

It is vitally important that people with learning disabilities have information that they can understand, about the positive aspects of sexual expression and relationships, and the need for safe sex. Therefore, support to people with learning disabilities to develop relationships needs the following elements:

- Families and supporters to reflect on their own value positions in relation to people with learning disabilities and sexuality.
- Services that are used by people with learning disabilities to have sexuality policies that can support them to express their sexuality and, if they wish, to form intimate relationships with others.
- To listen carefully to what people with learning disabilities want.
- To provide opportunities for people with learning disabilities to learn about sexuality and relationships in relevant and accessible ways.
- To view rights and 'protection' not as opposites but to seek ways in which people with learning disabilities can lead safe and fulfilling sexual lives.
- Accessible information and education about sexuality, feelings and relationships.

All these practical strategies are based on a rethink about the identity of 'having a learning disability', so that it can encompass the emotional and sexual needs that anyone has. Just as living independently does *not* mean doing everything for oneself, so too establishing a partner relationship can be done in the context of good support. For instance, a person with learning disabilities may wish to live together with their partner, either in a same-sex relationship or a heterosexual one. By doing that, they do not relinquish their need for support; instead, the planning for that support needs to take account of both partners, and any joint needs that they have. In most cases, that will result in a more efficient use of resources, but in any case, it will result in a lifestyle built on mutual love and trust, which is the most important part of anyone's life.

Supporting people with learning disabilities to be parents

Arguably the greatest challenge to services for people with learning disabilities is the idea that they too can be parents. The problem for social policy is a tension between the need to support parents with learning disabilities themselves, and the rights of their child to social protection. In general, the latter motive generally wins out (Kellett, 2011) since there is a responsibility on behalf of services to protect all children from abuse and neglect.

Nevertheless, support for many parents with learning disabilities can be structured so that they can be good parents (McConnell et al., 2010). Since 2005, a network of those who are interested in supporting parents with learning disabilities allows people to share and develop good practice in this area (Tarleton, 2012). For instance, a publication of stories of positive practice in supporting parents with learning disabilities concludes that support can be tailored to the particular learning styles and family needs of individuals. Despite the negative expectations and very real difficulties faced by these parents, they too can prove that they are effective and loving parents (see Resources section at end of chapter).

All parents need a range of supports when their children are young. People with learning disabilities too need support in order to parent well. However, poverty, lack of family support or lack of social networks may make obtaining support more difficult. In Iceland, Traustadottir and Sigurjonsdottir write positively of the experiences of parents with learning disabilities who are supported by their families and community. Their study of three families where people with learning disabilities were parents concluded that:

> Raising children involves a concerted effort by parents, extended family members, and community services and programs where the family usually plays the most important part. (Traustadottir and Sigurjonsdottir, 2010: 59–60)

Other research suggests the need for support from professionals that is long term, flexible (Guinea, 2001; O'Hara and Martin, 2003; Young and Hawkins, 2006) and well coordinated across different services (O'Hara and Martin, 2003). The kinds of support that parents may need will vary from one family to another and will also change over time. Tarleton et al. (2006) suggest some of the practical kinds of support that may be needed, which include support with actual child rearing skills, as well as support to themselves in managing finances and paperwork and coping with bullying or harassment. When interviewed, parents with learning disabilities also indicated a need for emotional support (Guinea, 2001). In part this seemed to be related to the narrower friendship network these parents had compared to parents in the general population.

Parents with learning disabilities at a national meeting in England outlined some of the things they felt would help them meet the challenges they faced in parenting. These are shown in Box 6.3.

Box 6.3	Parents: meeting the challenges

- Accessible information about their own health and the health of their baby and how to look after their baby.
- Self advocacy groups and coming together with other parents.
- Getting support before things go wrong and become a crisis.
- Being assessed in their own home, not in an unfamiliar residential family centre.
- Assessment and support by people who understand learning disabilities.
- Advocacy.
- Making courts accessible.
- Support for fathers.
- Support for women and men experiencing violent relationships.

Source: CHANGE, 2005, cited in Tarleton, 2010: 57

All of these challenges suggest the importance of partnerships and coordination of support as well as a recognition by service providers of the rights of people with learning disabilities to develop new identities, to contribute within relationships and to nurture future generations of children. Having access to good support services and forging new identities go hand in hand.

Conclusion: what has been achieved by new ways of seeing people with learning disabilities?

Relationships are central to how we see our own identity, and how others see us. For people with learning disabilities they are important both for supporting their inclusion in their communities and for moving towards the creation of a 'good life' (Johnson and Walmsley, 2010). However, the overriding message from this chapter is that the identity of 'learning disability' tends to dominate, and can easily create a stereotype of a person who cannot develop a deep or meaningful relationship. It is hoped that the individual voices and stories from this chapter help to counter that view, and to indicate the emotional depth and desires of people with learning disabilities. In developing that support, people with learning disabilities will be seen as individuals, in a new light – taking up roles such as friend, sexual partner, carer or parent. The evidence of this chapter seems to support the view that identity is a key concept, challenging the way people with learning disabilities are seen by others in society, and also how they see themselves.

The freedom to develop relationships can also be hampered, as seen in this chapter, because of concerns about risk and protection from harm. Those who provide social support to people with learning disability are guided not only by policies about autonomy, choice and control, but also by the need to protect vulnerable people from risk. In a risk-averse society, the duty of care can dominate in the relationship between a support provider and a person with learning disabilities. Recognizing people with learning disabilities as emotional and sexual beings is a challenge to many service providers and families. It is often seen as the polar opposite of providing good care and support, but this chapter suggests that the two aspects of identity support should be seen jointly. Teaching people about the nature of sexuality and finding ways to support them to lead good lives can also serve as a form of protection. By following up some of the good practice examples in the resource list below, readers may find some challenges and also some inspiration to think about 'learning disability' in a new way. The identity of 'learning disabled' has sometimes been referred to as stigmatized (see Goffman, 1963, for a discussion of the concept of stigma). The way in which people are viewed by others affects profoundly the way in which they think about themselves, as dependent on other more 'able' people to make the major decisions in their lives. If identity is socially constructed (De Fina *et al.*, 2006: 7), then that may imply that people with learning disabilities need to take up new roles, engage in different relationships, and encourage others to think about them in new ways (Williams, 2011). Perhaps the best way to reflect on these issues is to imagine one's own life without close personal relationships, and to consider how the view we have of ourselves can change, through the gaze of others who get to know us personally.

However, the conundrum still exists, that these are people who need support to manage everyday aspects of life. Can relationships be pursued independently, within that framework of support? Some very practical dilemmas can occur, where people are trying to develop personal, intimate relationships, with personal assistants present in the home. However, good support can be developed in respectful ways, as has for instance been demonstrated through the network of professionals working together with parents with learning disabilities (Tarleton *et al.*, 2006). Support issues will be explored further in Chapter 9, after the fundamental building block of person-centred planning that is the topic for the next chapter.

Reflection exercises

1. Identity may seem to be an obvious concept; it is simply about who we are, how we see ourselves and how others see us. There have been many theories of identity, and some of that range can be seen in the ESRC programme of studies, Identities and Social Action:

   www.open.ac.uk/socialsciences/identities

   Consider what methods you would use to explore identity issues with people with learning disabilities directly.

2. One of the best ways to consider relationships in the lives of people with learning disabilities is to contrast their situation with your own, or with other people you know. What relationships do you value in your own life, how did they come about, and how have they

changed how you see yourself? Reflect in a group discussion about the lives of particular people with learning disabilities, and how they contrast with your own.

3. Relationships and sexuality often fall outside the scope of funded support, but some would argue that social care policy can and must take account of the issues presented in this chapter, in order to ensure that people with learning disabilities are supported to have better relationships in their lives. Consider what professions should contribute jointly to an effective type of support service for some of the people whose views are represented in this chapter.

Suggested further resources

1. A list of resources for supporting parents with learning disabilities is given on the website of the Working Together with Parents Network. Other links on this website will also be useful for finding out more about parenting with support:

   www.bristol.ac.uk/wtwpn/resources/further-resources.pdf

2. The easy-information section of the Norah Fry Research Centre website includes two picture stories to promote discussion about same-sex relationships for people with learning disabilities ('Jan's Story' and 'Phil's Story')

   www.bristol.ac.uk/norahfry/easy-information

3. There are several websites being started up by dating agencies, or people with learning disabilities themselves who support each other to have better social lives. These include:

   http://stayuplate.org (a punk band 'with and without learning disabilities'); www.starsinthesky.co.uk (friendship and dating for people with learning disabilities).

7 Person-Centred Planning for Life

Moving into adulthood can be one of the most stressful times of life for anyone, and it poses particular challenges for people with learning disabilities. This chapter explores person-centred ways of approaching the period of 'transition to adulthood'.

Key points summary:

- Transition means becoming an adult. It is a word that is used to cover the move from children's services and school, into the things people want to do in adult life.
- Transition will only work well if people make good plans. That is why this chapter looks at person-centred planning at the time of transition.
- When people work in a person-centred way, that means that they are thinking about one person, and helping them to be in control of things. It is about helping someone to become the person they want to be.
- Person-centred planning is about what people are good at, and what they want in life. It is not just about needs and problems. It involves other people who can help a person to plan for their own life, in a practical way.
- But transition and planning can be used as an excuse. They will never work well unless there are good things for people to do, and support for them to live as adults.

Introduction and overview

> We make many transitions in our lives, but perhaps the one with the most far-reaching consequences is the transition into adulthood. (Heslop *et al.*, 2002)

'Transition' refers both to a period of time during which people are moving from childhood to adulthood, and also to a process by which transfer from children's to adult services takes place (Townsley *et al.*, 2004: 1). In all these transitions, this chapter will argue that the important issue is to ensure that the person with learning disabilities has a voice, has real options, and remains 'at the centre' of the plans for their own life. As with other chapters in this book, there is no intention of providing a comprehensive guide to practice; nevertheless this chapter in particular offers a strong link between policy and practice, namely person-centred planning (PCP). PCP methods are often referred to as a 'tool-box'. There are key references and information to follow up for practitioners at the end of the chapter, including the guide to person-centred approaches in transition planning, from the National Transition Support Team in the UK (see end of chapter).

A successful move into adult status for all young disabled people essentially involves a growth in self-determination, and an understanding of choice and control. The United Nations Convention on the Rights of the Child asserts the right of young people to be consulted about decisions affecting them, and, in the UK, the Children Act 1989 further enshrines this principle in law, explicitly extending it to young people with learning disabilities:

> Even children with severe learning disabilities or very limited expressive language can communicate preferences if they are asked in the right way … No assumptions should be made about 'categories' of children with disabilities who cannot share in decision-making. (vol. 6, para. 6.8)

However, gulfs can open up between words and action. The chapter will outline both the processes that are intended to ease transition, and the evidence about success of those processes. There appears to be a myriad of difficulties and barriers that have to be confronted at transition, and we will look at some examples of how these have been tackled, as well as the continuing problems for many young people and their families.

A young person with learning disabilities is not only faced with the challenge of growing up, and achieving the ordinary goals of all teenagers, such as relationships, fun, sex and financial independence, but is also faced with the job of learning how to exercise control over his or her own support services. Julian Goodwin's story at the start of Chapter 1 shows how all these elements of life are bound up with chance events and particularly with family circumstances. His move to America as a teenager only came about because of his father's job, although he did have some say in whether or not to move back to England subsequently. Throughout this chapter, I will take a broad view of transition as referring to a period of time, between the ages of 14 and 25, and I will try to highlight ways in which we can understand and challenge the barriers faced by young people with learning disabilities during that period of their lives. First I will examine the notion of person-centredness, before turning to the research literature about transition for young people with learning disabilities. Finally, this chapter will explore and reflect on some of the solutions in developing models of person-centred transition. As in other chapters in this book, the concept of person-centredness itself needs to be unravelled and questioned in more depth. That is what this chapter aims to do.

Key policy concept: person-centredness

Voice of Experience

I live with three other young people in a house with support in Essex. I moved there a few months ago. I left school last year and now I go to my local college, doing a life skills course. I am also doing a childcare course and spent time in a primary school. I want to keep fit so I go swimming three times a week. I really like having my hair styled every Thursday and having my nails painted.

I like meeting up with old school friends at a youth club every Thursday. I like being with small children and this is something I'd like to do after I leave college. I like being independent – doing housework like the washing and ironing and cleaning. I also like cooking Indian food and watching films with my housemates. I meet up with mum and dad every Sunday. I get scared and frightened of dogs. I also do not like insects so I need a lot of support if I see them.

Source: Melanie, aged 19, from 'We Can Dream', Davies *et al.*, 2011

What does 'person-centred' mean?

The question of what 'person-centred' actually means is intriguing. It would appear that the word has its origins in models of person-centred counselling. Carl Rogers's definition of working in a person-centred way involves the therapist in helping a person achieve their full potential as a human being:

> The goal the individual most wishes to achieve, the end which he knowingly and unknowingly pursues, is to become himself. (Rogers, 2004: 108)

This idea of knowing and supporting the individuality of a person is very relevant to the practice of person-centred planning (PCP). That is why Melanie, in the box above, was asked about what she likes doing, and what is important to her. In this context, the word 'person-centred' conveys a strong emphasis on the wishes and goals of the individual. For instance, the leading proponent of PCP in the UK claims that:

> Person centred planning assumes that people with disabilities are ready to do whatever they want as long as they are adequately supported. (Sanderson, 2000: 6)

Melanie, in the example above (Davies *et al.*, 2011), lived away from home. However, a circle of her friends and family worked on her person-centred plan with her, and Melanie was able to tell them that she really wanted to move back to the local area. One of the outcomes from her plan was that she did achieve that, but was also able to explore with her circle what support would suit her best. Melanie said that she really valued time away from her support-ers and friends, to have privacy. Through her person-centred plan, people have listened to her, and taken seriously what she felt about her life, and have helped her to move forwards.

Like so many of the terms in this book, using a word such as 'person-centred' represents an attempt to shift practice, recognizing that services and supports have not always operated by this principle. Planning for adult services, at its worst, can be dominated by bureaucratic, authoritarian styles of service provision, in which the service user is seen as the lowest part of the chain, accepting gratefully what is offered to him or her by society.

Person-centredness, then, is perhaps best understood by what it is not. In the lives of people with learning disabilities, there is a very deeply ingrained sense of professional control, which has a profound influence on how people see themselves. In an ongoing research study, a woman talking about her forth-coming assessment for social care was asked recently by the author what she wanted to get from it. After pausing for thought, she said: 'I really don't know. I'll wait and see – they will tell me.'

Working in a person-centred way with people with learning disabilities therefore often means facilitating someone and encouraging them, in order to overcome years of experience of being treated as less than equal, as needing control and guidance. Essentially it is about working in a way that respects the equality and humanity of each person, and establishing a relationship where they can start to become more aware of what they want to get out of life. That may mean setting aside the bureaucratic processes that tend to predominate in social and health care, so that, as Rogers wrote, the person can be allowed to 'become him or herself'.

Person-centred planning

Widely referred to in the development of policy and practice for people with learning disabilities in the UK, person-centred planning (PCP) was a recom-mendation of the Learning Disability White Paper, *Valuing People* (DH, 2001), and since then has been the cornerstone of the strategic agenda in learning disability and also in generic disability policy (PMSU, 2005). It is intended as a holistic process, which aims to ensure that the person with learning disabili-ties (focus person) is, as far as possible, in control of his or her life.

Originating from North American models (O'Brien *et al.*, 2000), PCP is intended to articulate the goals and wishes of the 'focus person' by enabling them to undertake in-depth planning of what is necessary to have the life they want (Sanderson *et al.*, 1999; Ritchie *et al.*, 2003; Routledge and Sanderson, 2002; O'Brien *et al.*, 2010). In the UK, these authors have had a profound influence on the way learning disability services and supports are shaped around the lives of individuals. They have made available both widespread PCP training, and the 'tools' for PCP and different models of PCP. These methods are often associated with visual means of recording, creative planning using different media, and with the notion of friends and family contributing their knowledge and building a picture of the young person's strengths, personality and particular preferences. In some forms of planning, such as Essential Lifestyle Planning (ELP), the emphasis is also on what *must* be in place to support someone, and the recording of the fine detail which so often makes the crucial difference between successful and unsuccessful support practices. As is frequently emphasized, PCP tools should not be seen simply as a menu. PATH planning, for instance, focuses on future goals, and the steps taken to move towards those goals, while other styles of planning may lead the person to reflect on their past experiences in order to plan for the future. However, a skilled facilitator can adapt and choose elements of different styles of planning as needed by a particular individual:

> Person centred planning is not simply a collection of new techniques for individual planning to replace previous approaches. It is based on new ways of seeing and working with people with disabilities, fundamentally about sharing power and community inclusion. (Sanderson, 2000: 2)

Melanie, in the example above, benefited because others took time to listen to her and find out what really mattered in her life. Most would agree with Mansell and Beadle-Brown (2004):

1. The concern of PCP is to reflect the unique circumstances of the individual.
2. PCP aims to consider aspirations and capacities, based on 'the authority of the service user's voice.
3. It attempts to include and mobilize the individual's family and wider social network; and
4. PCP gives support to achieve goals.

Planning within a personalized system of social care

While the moves towards PCP were developed largely with people with learning disabilities in the UK, more recently PCP has come to underpin a much wider system change in social care (Sanderson and Neil, 2009). Within a personalized model of social or health care, planning becomes a pre-requisite, and the support plan can drive resources and has a better chance of 'making something happen' at service level. A central tenet of personalization (see p. 21) is that the disabled person owns their own plan – in other words, that they have decided for themselves what goals are important to them, and what kind of support services will help them to achieve those goals. Planning out one's own support is central to personalization, for all service users, and research for the Office for Disability Issues (ODI) in England (Williams and Porter, 2011) examined how this happens, from the point of view of people with physical impairments, mental health needs, dementia and learning disabilities. In many respects, good support planning has all the features of person-centred planning, adapted to the needs and styles of individuals. In Williams and Porter (2011), the support planners felt that the central features of good support planning were about keeping the vision of self-directed support clear. It is the service user who is in charge, and who owns their own plan. The support planner therefore has in some ways a more subtle and sensitive role than a traditional manager. Their job is to open up people's ideas about 'what is possible' and to challenge people's perceptions of what they can do. In this study, it was found that this function could best be performed by disabled people's organizations, who were commissioned by the local authority to facilitate support plans. As with PCP, flexibility, creativity and trust were all seen to be essential: the support planner needs to take enough time to get to know what is important to the individual, and not simply slot them into services that are already there.

How then does this notion of support planning relate to PCP? Unfortunately, the proliferation of terminology is often matched by some confusion about different types of plans, and how they relate to each other. PCP can be seen as something separate and parallel, but not directly having the force of a support plan. For those who have personal budgets in England, the support plan has to be 'validated' by social services to ensure that the budget can be released and will be used in approved ways. Therefore a support plan is often seen as distinct from a PCP. Nevertheless, any form of personalized planning should contrast in significant ways with service planning led by an assessment of 'needs', and Brewster and Ramcharan (2005: 492–4) offer a useful point by point comparison of PCP with needs-led individual programme planning. In the end, these authors conclude that PCP is an evolutionary process, not a radical departure, from a wider movement towards individual autonomy:

> PCP is part of a wider move towards person–centred care that has increasingly come to characterize a central underlying value of human services within medical, health and social welfare. (Brewster and Ramcharan, 2005: 494)

The assumption in PCP is that an individual person with learning disabilities can achieve their goals, if they are supported by people who are really working together to ensure that the individual remains at the centre. Logically, this sounds like something that is ideally suited to planning at transition, and that is no doubt why the UK government (DH, 2001; 2009) has enthusiastically adopted the notion of person-centred planning within transition policy. Can PCP then turn around the experience of young disabled people at transition? The problems experienced at this stage are explored through research findings in the following section, before turning back to evidence about PCP as a potential catalyst for change.

Research about transition

Voice of Experience

I was mixed up between school and college. I wasn't in one head – I was in both … I change my mind all the time, but I want the support there when I want it. And I want to use it for whatever I want to use it for, and when I have finished with it, I put it back down. Friends are different – you can trust a friend with your secrets, even secrets you haven't told your parents. We can get stronger by supporting each other. It's helped me to control my anger, and to get a lot more confident about speaking up.

Source: young people in the 'Mind the Gap' research, in Jefferson *et al.*, 2006 (see Resource Section at end of chapter)

Relevant legislation and guidance about transition in England

Transition for young disabled people has received its fair share of attention in English policy documents and legislation, as summarized in Box 7.1. The process of transition has emerged both from educational policy and from policies relating to social care and health, as one of the central principles is that these services need to collaborate to assist young people at transition. Thus there are relevant aspects in policy for adult social care (for instance, the Direct Payments Act, 1996 and the extension of direct payments to 16- and 17-year olds in the 2001 Health and Social Care Act) which have an influence on young people's options.

There is a strong theme of the 'voice of the young person' which threads through these documents, urging professionals to step back, give good information and enable young people to speak up about their own goals in life. However, when young people themselves are asked about transition, they do not always come up with the key themes in policy. For instance, the young people in the 'Strongest Link' group whose viewpoints are given at the start of this section said that they wanted a trusted, familiar person to be there for them, who was always there when they wanted support. Other than that, they also placed a high value on friendship, and said that friends helped them with current problems and future plans.

Transition is not just about passing a disabled young person from one system to another; from 1996 onwards, transition review meetings have been tasked with considering all the key domains of young people's future lives, including education, employment, housing, health, transport and leisure. Nevertheless, there has also to be a strong emphasis on a systematic approach to transition planning. It is assumed that, with proper systems in place, the needs of all young people will be able to be met, if they are known about in good time. With that in mind, it is assumed that there is a need not only to get the transition process right for individual young people with learning disabilities, but also to plan strategically in local areas, and to know what services and supports are necessary for the future.

Box 7.1	Transition statements in English government policy

Legislation, guidance and government reports	Summary of how it relates to what should happen at transition
NHS Community Care Act 1990 and the Disabled Persons Act 1986	This legislation sets out the basis for the range of provision to disabled people (including children and young people). A mandatory link was introduced between education and social services so that the latter know about, and plan for, the needs of disabled children and young people.
Education Act 1996 and associated SEN Code of Practice (2001)	Requires any young person with a statement of special educational need (SEN) to have a transition plan drawn up by the local authority at the first annual statement review after they have started year 9. Details how the planning process should happen and key roles. Young people to be central and involved in the planning process. Should cover wide range of topics including development of autonomy and independence as well as self-advocacy.
Learning and Skills Act 2000	Creates an obligation to carry out assessments for young disabled people who plan to move on to further or higher education, or training. These assessments should form the basis of transition planning.
Health and Social Care Act 2001	Extends use of direct payments for disabled children and allows 16- and 17-year-olds to apply for a direct payment in their own right.
Valuing People 2001; Valuing People Now, 2009 (Strategies for Learning Disability, England); NSF: Children, Young People and Maternity Services, 2004; NSF Long term conditions, 2005	Charged Learning Disability Partnership Boards with identifying person with lead role on transition. Highlights need for continuity of support at transition for young people with learning disabilities. Standard 4 in the 2004 National Service Framework (NSF) covers transition and states that responsive, age appropriate services should be available as young disabled people move into adulthood. Standard 8 relates to transition for those with complex health needs and focuses on the process being person-centred and multi-agency.
Improving the Life Chances of Disabled People, 2005; Independent Living Review 2008 Transition: getting it right for young people, 2006 Transition: moving on well, 2008	Transition to adulthood one of four priority themes in 2005 report. Highlights need to focus on individual needs and wishes, as well as widening choice and transparency in transition planning. Recognizes the adverse effects of poorly planned transitions. Recommends ways of improving planning processes including holistic view of needs, recognizing individuality and additional needs of those with 'complex disability'. Good-practice examples.

Box 7.1 *Continued*

Legislation, guidance and government reports	Summary of how it relates to what should happen at transition
Aiming High for Disabled Children, 2007	Sets out the Transition Support Programme and £19m. available (2008–11) to promote consistently good practice, introduces 'core offer' to parents of disabled children which will be measured against a performance indicator. Core offer to be built around services performing well at: information, transparency, assessment, participation and feedback.

Adulthood is often a difficult concept for young people with learning disabilities and their families, since the traditional steps towards an independent adult life are not necessarily in place. Given that outcomes are, at best, problematic as young learning disabled people move into adulthood, the process of transition can be viewed simply as a smokescreen. Just like the words 'person-centred', transition itself may be a slippery term, something that distracts attention from the lack of substance, the problems for all young people with learning disabilities in becoming adults. It is possible to question the value of introducing yet another system, and paying attention to the meetings and plans in adolescence, rather than the provision of good options in adulthood.

The following sections will therefore summarize what that evidence is. What is known about the experiences young people with learning disabilities and their families have at the time of transition to adulthood?

Transition to adulthood: outcomes for young people and their families

A heavy policy emphasis on a particular topic generally signals that it is still problematic, and research has in fact consistently revealed the shortcomings of transition processes, both from the point of view of young people and of their families. For young people with learning disabilities, transition can be a very difficult time, as repeated studies have shown. There are many issues, and well-documented barriers, which are summed up here:

- Young people with learning disabilities simply do not have a large range of viable options for their future (Heslop *et al.*, 2002; Caton and Kagan, 2007; Davies and Beamish, 2009).
- The information needs of young people and their families are very seldom well met (Tarleton, 2004; Bhaumik *et al.*, 2011).
- The actual process of transition to adult status is often protracted, with traditional markers of adulthood not being met (Mitchell, 1999).
- Young people with learning disabilities are six times more likely than their

peers to develop mental health distress during this period (Emerson and Hatton, 2007b; Williams and Heslop, 2005).

A major multi-methods study of transition for young people with learning disabilities in the UK was carried out at the time of *Valuing People*, by Heslop *et al.* (2002). This study highlighted a number of areas where there were continuing problems in the implementation of official policy and guidance on transition, and concluded that for the majority of young people with learning disabilities and their families there was uncertainty, confusion and a lack of any real choice for the youngsters concerned. Problems related both to the process and the outcomes of transition. Ten years on, there are unfortunately still echoes of all these themes. A single case study of a local authority transition service (Tarleton and Porter, 2012) found that families of young people with learning disabilities still felt that they were fighting for services, and experienced adult services which were over-stretched and focusing on crisis work. The outcomes for young people in this study were bleak, with only one in eight obtaining any paid work, and others engaged in time-filling leisure activities. Despite some ten or more years of coor-dinated efforts to put in place policy for planned transitions, research is finding (Bhaumik *et al.*, 2011) that the same lack of planning, information and support is experienced by families of young people with learning disabilities in 2011 as in 2001. This is particularly acute for those families from minority ethnic groups. Transition planning also poses a particular difficulty for those who have moved away from their home area to attend residential schools and colleges. Heslop *et al.* (2007) found that parents valued having sufficient information, good forward planning, and said that they themselves often had to be proactive and to foster good connections with other parents, in order to achieve a good outcome for their son or daughter who was returning from residential school.

These themes unfortunately have echoes around the world. For instance, Davies and Beamish (2009), in a survey of 218 parents of young people with learning disabilities in Australia, reported that their lives were profoundly affected by changes to the family at 'transition' and mothers were often forced to give up work at that point in order to provide adequate care. As one parent in this study said, finishing school for a child with SEN can be 'like falling off a cliff ... a huge void' (Davies and Beamish, 2009: 255).

Young people with learning disabilities do not just seek 'adult services'. Particularly over the years since 2009, paid employment has resurfaced as a valued policy goal for all people with learning disabilities. This is also so in Australia, where Winn and Hay (2009) found that successful transition to work was associ-ated with a positive work ethic and identity among young people with learning disabilities and their families, as well as work experience at school age. However, these authors found a disjointed and fragmented service provision for people with learning disabilities in adulthood, coupled with prejudice against disabled people in the workplace. Similarly, Kaehne's (2010) content analysis of Welsh local authority protocols for school to 'workplace' transitions showed that they were widely discrepant and not always effective in communicating with other agencies, let alone with the people themselves who are at the centre of the transition.

However good the process of transition, clearly a lack of viable options post-school is the main obstacle for most young people with learning disabilities.

Whose voice counts at transition?

Compared with the evidence about outcomes, there is less about the *process* of transition, despite the plethora of guidance. The 2001 SEN Code of Practice underlines the fact that 'the views of young people themselves should be sought and recorded wherever possible' during any review or assessment (SEN Code of Practice, 9:55). This document also details the support that might be necessary, in order to achieve that goal. This includes the provision of accurate information to the child, support to the child in the form of a known person such as a learning support assistant, the use of an advocate and full explanation to the child about the role of other professionals involved in the transition process. Yet Heslop *et al.* (2002) found that only 12 out of 27 young people with learning disabilities interviewed about their transition meetings felt that they had been given any choices about what they wanted to do after leaving school. Half of all the young people had attended a planning meeting, but only two-fifths of those had directly contributed their views during a meeting. As Heslop *et al.* (2002) put it, 'attendance had not (always) meant engagement'.

More recently, research has explored in greater detail how these shortcomings at transition are played out in the course of interactions during meetings. Pilnick *et al.* (2010, 2011) are among the few authors to examine transition planning using the methodology of conversation analysis (CA), and their data on the whole lend weight to the problematization of transition planning. By analysing the fine-grained detail of interactions in transition-planning meetings, Pilnick *et al.* showed how professionals and parents used strategies which created young people's goals as 'unreasonable' (Pilnick *et al.*, 2011: 318). This highlights the dilemma at the heart of any group decision-making process, namely the difficulty of attributing a decision to one individual. Pilnick *et al.* (2010) analysed how young people's contributions and voice could be sidelined in the course of the interaction, with the agenda being strongly set by the need to determine educational goals for future college placements. When asked therefore about their future goals, a young person might say they wanted to 'do painting' or 'be a policeman'. Pilnick *et al.* (2010: 424) showed how these responses could be *interactionally* relevant (i.e. they fitted within what was expected of a young person, in terms of speaking up in their transition review). However, at the same time they could be worked up as 'contextually problematic', since they were not within the range of answers considered appropriate for planning a college course.

In a study carried out in partnership with a self-advocacy group for people with learning disabilities, Tarleton (2004) also found that parents explained their frustration about transition in ways that resonate with Pilnick *et al.*'s findings. Parents frequently felt the hollowness of the status of adulthood at the age of 18, when they said they were left making key decisions and guiding the life of the young person with learning disabilities in their family. Not only did they feel that they still held that responsibility, but they were also frustrated by their formal lack of a voice. While their son or daughter was still at home, the parent role moved into one of 'carer', and there are at least some rights for carers under UK policy. However, when the young person moved away from the home, the parent could feel even more cut off in terms of role and status:

> Now he's over 21, in supported living, I feel excluded, I don't have any involvement in decisions. (Tarleton, 2004)

Pilnick *et al.*'s (2010: 433) analysis showed how an attempt to be empowering could paradoxically end in an undermining of choice and control, and Clegg *et al.* (2008) discuss data from the same study, concluding on the basis of parents' narratives that individual decision making and autonomy should not be the mantra at transition, and that:

> [we] need to … shift the moral compass away from individual achievement and towards engagement and relationships. (Clegg *et al.*, 2008: 93)

A dilemma no doubt exists, when trying to promote autonomy and ensure that the individual young person truly has a say in their own future. In this context, can a person-centred approach, and the use of PCP in particular, make a difference?

Person-centred planning in practice

Examples of person-centred approaches

 Voice of Experience

The sky's the limit, in terms of what someone wants to do with their life. Chris wants to make computer games, and to do that he needs to go to college to study science and maths. At the moment, he loves school, and he has lots of friends. There are people to enrol in his life, to make sure they help him get to his goals. They can write their names on his plan. Chris' assistant at school says: 'A next step may be for Chris to get an apprenticeship when he leaves school, so that he can work on computers. And that way he'll earn money, which is also something he wants to do. The apprenticeship my son's on pays him £80 a week. And he could get support from direct payments.' Chris' mum says: It's very rewarding, that so many people want to help Chris, and the same people are going to be involved in the future – not just dropping out as time goes by.

Source: Helen Sanderson Associates *et al.*, 2010

How can a young person with learning disabilities be well supported to move into adulthood, to 'get a life'? This is the name of an initiative in the UK, in which a number of demonstration sites explored how partnership between local agencies can assist young people to develop their own, holistic, plans and put them into action. The example above is taken from a DVD produced by policy makers and development organizations in England, showing how transition can be an ordinary experience, involving family and friends. The DVD is divided into the six steps for achieving citizenship (Duffy, 2003), namely self-determination, self-direction, money, home, support and community. The message is that we should never assume that young people cannot speak up for themselves: with sufficient support, youngsters with learning disabilities can say what they want, and can be helped to achieve their goals.

Accounts of the PCP process by people with learning disabilities themselves (e.g. Clark et al., 2005) are invariably positive, focusing on the greater sense of security, involvement, and confidence brought by the social support offered by others. Indeed, these accounts frequently emphasize the social and relational nature of decision making in PCP, and the benefits it brings. As Doris Clarke says in her story, she especially enjoyed meeting her circle of friends at the pub, or going out for meals and other social events (Clark et al., 2005).

The transition process is not just about meetings, and of course young people with learning disabilities can make their views known in other ways. Innovative practices can include video diaries, taster days at local colleges, or photographic records of people's own plans (see end of chapter). Particularly for those with profound learning disabilities, and severe communication difficulties, decision making has to be within a social context. For instance, Vlaskamp et al. (2009) in the Netherlands describe a system of individualized support planning for people with profound and multiple learning difficulties (PMLD), which focuses on 'perspectives'. These are long-term goals which are set by family and friends who know the person well. However, these authors found in their study of one residential facility that short-term goals to back up the 'perspective' for each client were not always in place. The practical steps are perhaps more difficult to put in place, compared with the overall aspiration for each person.

Although we can critique and pull apart the practices and principles underlying individual autonomy and choice-making by young people with learning disabilities, nevertheless there is a certain value base underpinning PCP and person-centred practice which is undeniable. Readers will find many more examples by following the leads at the end of this chapter. As Gurit et al. (2010: 112) maintain, basic ethical practice includes adopting 'a moral principle of respect for persons [with learning disability]'), and therefore PCP appears to be reasonably uncontroversial, in setting out a practical way for engaging families and communities, along with service providers, with the person with learning disabilities 'at the centre' and in control. We will turn now to evidence about its success in achieving outcomes.

The outcomes of person-centred planning

The first and major evidence base for PCP in England is a study of four sites in England, where 93 people with learning disabilities were moved over to a PCP model (Robertson *et al.*, 2005, 2007a). On most measures, PCP was shown to be beneficial, and for people with learning disabilities 'modest positive changes' were found in the areas of social networks; contact with family; contact with friends; community-based activities; scheduled day activities; and choice (see also Mansell and Beadle-Brown, 2004; Cambridge *et al.*, 2006).

The same study by Robertson *et al.* in 2005 has given rise to several further analyses. For instance, Robertson *et al.* (2007a) report on a multivariate factor analysis to discover what factors were associated with improved outcomes for people with learning disabilities. Summing together some of the individual factors that were systematically investigated in this analysis, it seemed that 'the commitment of facilitators to PCP' was the most powerful predictor of whether people would receive a plan, and was also related to increased chances of benefiting' (Robertson *et al.*, 2007a: 241). The benefits listed included contact with friends, social networks and hours per week of activity. However, there were found to be inequalities embedded in the chances of people having these benefits in the first place, since these authors found that those with autism and additional psychiatric disabilities were less likely to have a PCP.

Based on the same study, Robertson, Hatton *et al.* (2007b) analysed questionnaires, which were completed every three months by a variety of 'key informants' associated with the 93 people who had person-centred plans. Barriers to implementing PCP were found to include the lack of availability of trained facilitators, a lack of services, lack of time and reluctance of people other than paid support staff to engage in the PCP process. In order to ensure that PCP works, therefore, ongoing training and support for PCP facilitators are clearly needed.

Finally, Wigham *et al.* (2008) analysed the open comments from key informants in the Robertson *et al.* (2005) research. Reports of the benefits of PCP included increased activities and opportunities, the chance to take a fresh look at the person and their life, and the fact that the person themselves felt that they had more control and choice – according to Wigham *et al.* (2008) people with learning disabilities generally felt more confident and happier after having a PCP. The introduction of PCP brought with it a 'flurry of activity' around each person, which tended to have immediate benefits, whether or not these were sustainable in the longer term.

The UK research is therefore broadly positive in tone, and is matched by similar results about outcomes from PCP from a study in Ireland (McCormack and Farrell, 2009). In Ireland, a balanced picture was obtained from quality-of-life measures, appearing to show that PCP did lead to better outcomes in realizing personal goals, privacy and contact with loved ones, although people still did not achieve some basic rights, such as choosing where to live, and it was hardest to get good outcomes for people with PMLD (McCormack and Farrell, 2009). Further, there is evidence from an EU project (Lunt and Hinz, 2011: 14) that PCP is developing throughout Europe, albeit at different rates, and an evidence base is beginning to grow. For instance, German research has focused on evaluation of training programs for PCP facilitators, and in Sweden, the right to a person-centred plan is mandated by law (Lunt and Hinz, 2011: 13).

Can person-centred approaches achieve systemic change?

There is thus limited but positive evidence that a person-centred planning-process helps young people with learning disabilities achieve some better outcomes than they would otherwise have done. However, research has also revealed some of the difficulties and barriers faced by authorities in changing the 'system' of allocating care. Dowling *et al.* (2007) provide a useful review of research relating to PCP, based on a systematic search of the literature prior to 2007. The review revealed systemic barriers which hinder the progress of PCP, barriers which lay in the way support services were commissioned and funded. There were also barriers identified by research about the service infrastructure and the culture of services, that were often at odds with the ethos of person-centred planning. Staff need time and training to carry out person-centred planning, to understand the essential differences between PCP and previous forms of planning, and also to surrender control over what happens in people's lives.

The research also revealed some positive trends, with policy encouragement towards PCP, and service development being key supportive factors. The development of guidance (Routledge *et al.*, 2002) and also training for all parties involved in PCP (Coyle and Maloney, 1999) emerged as most helpful, although the authors admit that PCP depends to some extent 'on community and social networks that are supportive'. Therefore wider social barriers have to be addressed (Dowling *et al.*, 2007: 79). O'Brien *et al.* (2010) in fact see person-centred planning as a basis for building communities, not just services.

Much depends of course on the way in which service providers, assessors and local authorities can reconfigure their own roles and take a wider view of support for people with learning disabilities, as Cole and Williams (2007) discovered in their review of the changing nature of day opportunities for people with learning disabilities (see Chapter 10). Williams and Battleday (2007) in a study of care planning in the south-west of England, also found that systemic, creative solutions were possible when person-centred plans were implemented and listened to by local planners and commissioners. For instance, in one case, four young people with profound and multiple learning disabilities were returning from residential colleges, and their families worked with the local authority to establish a house where all four could live together, with flexible, individual support arrangements. As Dowling *et al.* concluded in 2007, research broadly does support the notion that it is possible to change services through and towards a PCP approach:

> A service culture that embraces ideas of empowerment and inclusion, is open to possibilities, willing to take risks and think outside traditional planning models, is therefore likely to facilitate person centred planning. (Dowling *et al.*, 2007: 79).

Since these research studies about PCP, the major thrust in England and Wales has been towards personal budgets (see Chapter 2, pp. 21–2). As mentioned above, research has started to investigate how that type of planning works best, and how styles of planning can best be suited to different individuals (Williams and Porter,

2011). Participants in that research appreciated particularly a support planner who did not simply *listen* to what they might say they want. The support planner who was most appreciated was someone who challenged people to think beyond their immediate aspiration, and to see what might be possible, and was then able to help them flesh that out into real packages of support (e.g. personal assistance, activities, living arrangements, aids and adaptations). As one participant in that study put it, the ideal facilitator was:

> [Someone who] would write down what you said, and then they would pull apart what you said, to get deeper into what you want, and what you're thinking and what you're saying. (Williams and Porter, 2011: 46)

Support planning sounds very similar, in the experience of these participants, to person-centred planning, being distinguished by informality, peer advice and support, listening skills, and facilitation for the disabled person to remain in control of their own support services. The question in 2012 is whether this more widespread notion of support planning can remain intact, without being drawn back into local authority mechanisms and bureaucracy.

Conclusion: what has person-centred transition planning achieved?

The policy concept explored in this chapter has proved perhaps the most uncontroversial yet. Working in a 'person-centred' way has a warm ring to it, like the idea of 'partnership' in Chapter 5, and 'inclusion' in Chapter 4. However, compared with those other policy goals, the advantage of person-centredness is that the policy rhetoric is matched by a practice tool, namely person-centred planning. The evidence from research has revealed that person-centred planning (PCP) can achieve beneficial outcomes for at least some people with learning disabilities, and the ethos of PCP is currently mirrored by the goals of support planning for all disabled people who use personal budgets.

Nevertheless, the particular period of transition to adulthood remains problematic for young people with learning disabilities and their families, and the review of research in that area proved rather depressingly constant in its messages about lack of provision, lack of information and support services. However person-centred the *process* of transition becomes, the outcomes can only be good if there are sufficient opportunities for people with learning disabilities to lead a fulfilling life in adulthood. Some of the problems and issues relating to housing in particular will be explored in the following chapter. For the moment, however, it should be noted that the term 'transition' can be used as a smokescreen, allowing a focus on the *process* of transition planning, at the expense of the provision of good options for the future.

PCP processes themselves have also been criticized, as has been explored in this chapter. For instance, there is criticism among some researchers and scholars (Clegg *et al.*, 2008) about the notion of individuality contained within PCP and indeed within personalized systems of social care. When PCP processes are shown to run counter to the choices articulated by people with learning disabilities, some authors argue that decision making is always going to be difficult for people with learning disabilities:

> ID is more than a social construct; it is also an embodied reality, which affects the ability of individuals to make rational autonomous decisions. (Pilnick *et al.*, 2010: 305)

Clegg *et al.* (2008) argue further that it is time to turn back from the individual towards the collective provision of support services. Similarly, there could be tensions between PCP and the idea of political, social change (Roulstone and Prideaux, 2012: 103). Is policy at risk of setting out to work on individuals, rather than on social barriers?

From the evidence in this chapter, it would seem important therefore to refocus on the meaning of person-centredness. Like all the concepts explored in this book, the word can become overused and devalued. However, using person-centred approaches at transition is not *just* about enabling an individual to articulate their own goals and dreams. That is certainly the basis of the philosophy, but, as seen in this chapter, PCP is about mobilizing communities, friendship circles and families and is also about engaging with system change and those who are paid to put into place support services. While the personalized aspect of transition is essential, nevertheless it is important that planners and managers in all agencies take on individual information and plan ahead for services and supports. It is only with a systematic and strategic approach that the opportunities for young people will actually exist when they leave the formal education system. The outcomes of person-centred plans, for instance, can and should be discussed at local authority level, since they may affect the types of commissioning which will be possible and necessary for the future. However person-centred we become at an individual level, nothing will ever really change until there are systemic shifts, more resources, more opportunities and changes in attitude.

Reflection exercises

1. Sometimes a particular concept can spawn a whole movement for change, and it may be that person-centred planning will be seen historically as one of those moments of change. It is interesting to review the evidence given in this chapter, and to find more international examples (see Resources section below), in order to discuss why PCP has had such an effect.

2. PCP brings together practical tools for change, with a philosophy that is intrinsically about our shared humanity. It seems to have a high chance of success in changing service cultures in the UK. However, the problems at transition are perhaps not about the

quality of planning, but about the outcomes and the lack of positive opportunities for people with learning disabilities as adults. Reflect with others on how PCP can be used to bring about systemic changes (see also FPLD website given below), and identify what professions would need to be involved and how practitioners can work together to achieve systemic change.

3. Both transition and person-centred planning can be seen as smokescreens or delaying mechanisms. Think of transition from the point of view of a person with learning disabilities, such as Melanie in the example on p. 116. What matters to her, and can a person-centred approach really make a difference to her life?

Suggested further resources

1. To learn more about the practices and tools of PCP, the best place to start is Helen Sanderson's website (HSA):

   www.helensandersonassociates.co.uk

2. The origins of PCP and a detailed, practical rationale can be found within the books which outline the American approach, and those which drew on that approach in the UK, for instance:

   Mount, Beth (1992) *Person-Centred Planning: A Sourcebook of Values, Ideas and Methods to Encourage Person-Centred Development*, New York: Graphic Futures.
   Sanderson, H., Kennedy, J., Ritchie, P. and Goodwin, G. (1997) *People, Plans and Possibilities: Exploring Person Centred Planning*, Edinburgh: SHS.

3. Taking PCP into practice, developing plans, and pushing for systemic change have all been part of the work done at the Foundation for People with Learning Disabilities (FPLD). Just explore their website to find out more: www.learningdisabilities.org.uk

4. Guidance about transition in England and Wales for young people with learning disabilities can be found on the Department of Health website: www.dh.gov.uk

5. The National Transition Support Team (2011) has lots of information, including *Person Centred Approaches in Transition Planning*:

www.transitioninfonetwork.org.uk/pdf/NTST_Person_Centred_
Approaches.pdf

6. The 'Strongest Link' pack was made for young people, by other
   young people with learning disabilities. It is available at:

   www.learningdisabilities.org.uk/publications

8 Making Decisions about where to Live

People with learning disabilities in England are among the very few groups of adults who do not regularly have a chance to choose who they live with. That is why this chapter links the notions of capacity and autonomy with evidence about housing options. This chapter explores decision making about where to live, with a particular focus on the Mental Capacity Act 2005 (MCA 2005) in England and Wales.

Key points summary:

- People with learning disabilities have a right to make decisions, and to have support for decisions. Everyone makes choices with some help from other people.
- People with learning disabilities have often lived in places where they can get support and care. But that can mean they themselves have little choice about where to live, and who to live with.
- Mental capacity law means that people can have others help them make decisions, but also others can make decisions for them in their best interests. They should only do that if the person cannot manage to understand and make the decision themselves.
- People do not always stay in one home. As people with learning disabilities get older, support services should think about each person's changing needs. Different types of support services need to link up more closely.

Introduction and overview

In the quotation on the top of page 134, Angela reflects on the fact that she finds her fellow residents 'a bit noisy'. Her life, like those of others where she lives, depends largely on the skills and good will of the staff. The house in which she lives is totally identified with the provision of support, and that is so for many people with learning disabilities. Therefore she has had little say about who her fellow residents would be, and this violation of choice was highlighted by people with learning disabilities as a research priority (Williams *et al.*, 2008b) and is also a priority for policy (DH, 2009d).

Voice of Experience

How do you feel about where you are living?

It's alright, a bit noisy. One person there is not a very nice person, but most of them are friendly. If people do something wrong, they get told off. The staff are sometimes very good, and know the things I want to do or buy. They do think of me. But to go out to the shops, I need two staff to be 'on'. They often don't have enough staff. I like living there, not because of the house. But I like it because I can go to People First.

Source: 'Angela' [not real name], in conversation with author, 2010

The decision to move house or to set up home with someone else is very central to the lives of most citizens in England and Wales. In fact, those who may lack capacity to make these decisions are now protected by law, and have rights to be supported, to have their capacity assessed, and to be involved in a person-centred way in decisions about their lives. Therefore, this chapter will start by giving a brief overview of the Mental Capacity Act 2005 (MCA 2005), the legal framework in England and Wales about supporting decisions, and enabling people to be at the heart of decisions made on their behalf. The ability to make a decision strikes at the heart of what it means to have a learning disability. On the one hand, it is often assumed that people with that label will not be responsible enough to make far-reaching decisions about their lives, while on the other hand, choice and control are the mantras of social care policy, as was seen in Chapter 2.

Moving house is often a complex and difficult decision to make, and one which affects not only the person with learning disabilities, but also his/her family, and others supporting him or her. Therefore, moving house represents one of the larger, more contentious issues for people with learning disabilities. The central part of this chapter continues by offering an overview of research about housing options, historical trends in institutional living, and the move to 'the community'. The majority of people with learning disabilities (at least 50 per cent in the UK, according to Emerson *et al.*, 2005) have always lived at home with their parents; in many other countries, there have never been alternatives to the family home. The issues facing families were discussed in Chapter 5, but their contribution and centrality to all the chapters cannot be emphasized enough. As with many non-disabled people, it is common to refer to the parental home as 'home', even when the person has moved away and set up their own place some time previously.

Given that people with learning disabilities do grow up, have a right to move on and to establish their own lives separately from their parents, there is always going to be an issue about housing and support provision which enables that move to happen. Julian, in his story at the start of Chapter 1, was fortunate to have already moved into a flat which he owned, before he started living more independently. Others may pursue options such as shared ownership or specific schemes for housing, if they want to have their own place. In countries other than the UK, finding a house or flat is sometimes an almost insuperable problem, and in many European countries, people with learning disabilities may find themselves in institutions, once their parents are no longer able to support them at home. This chapter will discuss some of the background in housing policy and practice, as well as current routes for people with learning disabilities to find 'a place to call home'.

In the final part of the chapter, the themes of decision making and housing will be brought together, through a summary of research about the MCA, in relation to changes of accommodation. This will particularly highlight the right of people with learning disabilities to remain at the centre of decisions that affect their interests. It should be noted that, while the MCA applies only to England and Wales, capacity legislation elsewhere (e.g. the Adults with Incapacity (Scotland) Act 2000) is based on similar principles. For instance, both the MCA and the Scottish Act enshrine the right of a person *with capacity* to make unwise decisions, and both treat capacity as specific to each decision. This chapter will conclude with some discussion about the tensions and challenges facing people with learning disabilities today, in their quest both for autonomy and for options about where to live.

Key policy concept: mental capacity and decision making

Autonomy

> People want to have more control of their own health, as well as their care. There is solid evidence that care is less effective if people feel they are not in control. A fundamental aim is to make the actions and choices of people who use services the drivers of improvement. They will be given more control over – and will take on greater responsibility for – their own health and well-being. (DH, 2006: 1.5)

One of the major goals of support services in Western welfare states in the twenty-first century is for individual service users to have greater autonomy in decisions about the support services they may need. This notion, sometimes referred to as 'personalization' (see Chapter 2, p. 21) has been the backdrop throughout this book, but it poses both opportunities and challenges for people with learning disabilities. Within a personalized model of social and health care (see Chapter 2, pp. 21–2), decisions are situated as close as possible to the service user. Decisions need to be made about education, family life, housing, work, health and day activities. This chapter will focus particularly on issues to do with decisions about where to live.

Statements such as the one above from English health and social care policy imply a more person-centred way of working than has been common previously in social services or health bureaucracies. Beyond that, they imply a situation in which individual 'service users' can be trusted, as autonomous human beings, to decide for themselves what they want, to take responsibility and to control their own services and supports (Beresford, 2001). The notion of individual autonomy is much cherished in Western societies, but does not entirely match the evidence about decision making, particularly with people with learning disabilities. This chapter will pose questions about collective, as well as individual, decisions.

Supporting mental capacity

Voice of Experience

A woman with learning disabilities who talked about her life to the author was 'Jane'. She was 35 and had lived with her father most of her life. She did have a short period of living in a 'training' hostel, but this did not work out for her. She was now living back with her dad. She said she is 'not impressed' with where she lives, since it is a rough area. However, she would rather live with her dad until she finds a place of her own. When asked about the future, she said that if she had to move anywhere, she would like to be in the countryside rather than town. She would like to live with friends.

Decision making and autonomy have been the focus of debate and interest among practitioners in England and Wales, both before and since the passing of the MCA, which came into force in 2007. In many countries, including the Netherlands (Wagemans *et al.*, 2010) and the USA (Adler, 2010), there is legislation that governs the issues of capacity to make decisions, and in most cases laws are designed to give protection to those who cannot make decisions for themselves. However, the English MCA has some significant differences from other international models, and has been described as 'personalized' capacity legislation.

Prior to 2007, capacity was generally assessed in an informal way, with an emphasis on the 'common sense' view that carers and family members could and should speak for the individual, particularly in more complex matters relating to health, finance or housing (Shah, 2010). However, since the MCA, the practices surrounding supported decision making and capacity have been clarified in England and Wales. The five basic principles of the MCA are given in Box 8.1.

Thinking of the story of 'Jane' above, the first three of these principles would imply that she should be supported to make her own decision. They specify that there should be, in all cases, a presumption of capacity – i.e. that Jane should not be considered to lack capacity, simply on the grounds of a learning disability. Instead, people should try to assess whether she understands enough to make the decision with support. They also mention the 'practical steps' that may need to be taken, to support a person to make their decision, and they even specify the right anyone has to make an 'unwise decision'. In other words, just because others may

Box 8.1	The five principles of the Mental Capacity Act 2005 (England and Wales)

1. A person must be assumed to have capacity unless it is established that he lacks capacity.
2. A person is not to be treated as unable to make a decision unless all practicable steps to help him to do so have been taken without success.
3. A person is not to be treated as unable to make a decision merely because he makes an unwise decision.
4. An act done, or decision made, under this Act for or on behalf of a person who lacks capacity must be done, or made, in his best interests.
5. Before the act is done, or the decision is made, regard must be had to whether the purpose for which it is needed can be as effectively achieved in a way that is less restrictive of the person's rights and freedom of action.

judge that Jane's wish to move to the countryside is unwise, that does not in itself mean that she lacks capacity. This is one of the aspects of the MCA which causes the greatest concern to those who support people with learning disabilities, and there is a fine line between a lack of capacity to *make* a decision and a lack of capacity to make the *right* decision, as will be explored later.

The principles involved in supporting decisions are underlined in the Code of Practice to the MCA (DH, 2007), and include the necessity to include the person who lacks capacity, as far as is possible, to communicate in accessible ways, to give time for the person to relax and think about the decision, and to have support from people they trust.

Box 8.2	Mental Capacity Act guidance on supporting decisions

The Act requires that before assessing a person as lacking capacity, all practical steps must be taken to support the person to make the decision for themselves. These steps are summarized in the Act's Code as follows:

- Using a different form of communication (for example non-verbal communication).
- Providing information in a more accessible form (for example, photographs, drawings, or tapes).
- Treating a medical condition which may be affecting the person's capacity.
- Having a structured programme to improve a person's capacity to make particular decisions (for example, helping a person with learning disabilities to learn new skills).

Source: DCA, 2007: 22

Best interests decisions

Despite the emphasis on supported autonomy, there are times when a person with learning disabilities may not be able to understand enough to make a decision and communicate it to others. At this point, again, under English law, it is normally not necessary to call in a psychologist or another specialist to assess capacity: anyone who is involved with the decision can and should assess the individual's capacity. For instance, in the case of a medical decision, this is likely to be the doctor or nurse. In the case of a decision about moving house, this might be family members, a social care practitioner or even a housing association officer. Assessment of capacity is intended to be a relatively informal affair, geared entirely to the particular decision being made. There is clear guidance that the presumption should be firstly that a person *has capacity* for the decision to be made, and the assessment should expressly *not* be influenced by the person's appearance or status as a person with a learning disability. Instead, an assessor should ask:

■ Does the person have a general understanding of what decision they need to make and why they need to make it?
■ Does the person have a general understanding of the likely consequences of making, or not making, this decision?
■ Is the person able to understand, retain, use and weigh up the information relevant to this decision?
■ Can the person communicate their decision (by talking, using sign language or any other means)?
■ Would the services of a professional (such as a speech and language therapist) be helpful?

If a person clearly cannot understand, weigh up or communicate information they need in relation to a particular decision in their life, then the 'best interests' principle is put into practice. The guiding points in making a best interests decision are that people should still be encouraged to participate in their own decision, but that the 'best interests decision maker' should find out as much as possible about what the person would have wanted, by consulting others who know him or her. Additionally, they should avoid discrimination, and not make assumptions about someone's best interests because of their 'age, appearance, condition or behaviour'. A full list of points is given in the MCA Code of Practice: section 5:65.

In the case of a person with learning disabilities moving house, the logic is that support should be offered first, to ensure that the person understands as far as possible what is going on. In a story such as Jane's mentioned above, it is frequently the case that the family member becomes unable to support Jane any longer, or Jane herself starts to feel she'd like to move on. Jane should not simply be 'moved out' into a group home or into some other housing. The first step should always be information, explanation and exploration of Jane's views, whether or not Jane has the ability to really make that decision by herself. However, it should be noted that none of this implies that Jane has a right to stay put, and that her relative's wishes are overlooked. If there is a *need* to move out of the parental home, then Jane's choices are effectively between other possible accommodation options.

Although the MCA makes a distinction between supported decisions and best interests decisions, nevertheless, the principles about listening and involving an individual are very similar, whether or not a person is deemed to lack capacity. However, where previously it was assumed that a family member or carer would speak *for* the person with learning disabilities at major turning points in their life, now there is a structure which should ensure either that the person is supported to make their own decision, or that a 'decision maker' leads a process to weigh up a person's best interests. While family members and others will still be consulted, it is quite possible that their views may contradict the best interests of the person with learning disabilities. However, in practice, research has found that decision makers will go a long way to avoid these conflicts, and to seek reconciliation and consensus (Williams *et al.*, 2012). This raises questions about the whole notion of individual autonomy, as it may be argued that all these decisions are effectively joint, collective affairs. Some would argue that this is no different from social decisions for anyone, which are seldom a private or individual affair. These issues, and models of best interests decisions, will be explored further after an exploration of the research evidence about housing options.

Research about housing options

Changes in policy and practice

How can people with learning disabilities best be supported, so that they have some choice about where they live? This question has often been phrased in a different way, without much room for personal decisions. Over the whole of the twentieth century, as Emerson (2005: 109) maintains: 'An important question for societies and their public agencies … has been what type of accommodation should be provided to those people with learning disabilities for whom neither independent living nor family support is an option'. The answer that has been given to that simple question has guided the direction of whole eras of practice, having a profound influence on the lives of people with learning disabilities.

In England, the 2001 Learning Disability strategy, *Valuing People*, did not take a very strong line on housing policy. The key actions mentioned in 2001 included joint working between housing and social services at local level, the prioritization of 'supported living' (see below) and the need to close the remaining long-stay hospitals. However, housing was a priority for action in the renewed strategy *Valuing People Now* (DH, 2009a). Concurrently, Townsley *et al.* (2009) in an analysis of independent living strategy and practice across Europe, identified that, with a few notable exceptions, people with learning disabilities were nearly always the ones who were left out of the moves towards independent living. Underpinning this are two tensions:

- **Competence and autonomy**: are people with learning disabilities restricted from making their own decisions because they are presumed to be 'incompetent'?
- **Risks and safety**: if we encourage people to move into the community and do 'ordinary' things that we all want to do, will that put them in danger?

Segregated, congregate models of living

Until the late 1980s and 1990s, people with learning disabilities normally moved out of the family home straight to some form of institution. Walmsley (1999) attributes the institutional movement to the twin goals of society to provide 'care', while asserting 'control', and in fact protecting the general population from any contact with those at its margins. Chapter 2 included some detail about the history of institutional practices, to which we do not need to return now.

The closure of institutions across Northern Europe and also in North American countries was driven by new moves towards 'normalization' (Nirje, 1969; Wolfensberger, 1972), a concept also discussed in Chapter 2 of this book. At the root of normalization was the notion that people's lifestyle should resemble as closely as possible the norms that non-disabled people value for themselves. However, this does not uniquely lead to one housing option over another. In the UK there is now a growing range of housing options and models of support, as was shown in Emerson *et al.*'s survey in 2005. Nevertheless, half of the respondents were still living with parents, and a further 12 per cent with other relatives, and 19 per cent were in residential care. The options of supported living, living alone or with a partner accounted for only 18 per cent of people with learning disabilities in England and Wales in 2004/5.

Although residential institutions have been largely discredited in the UK, partly because of widespread abuse revealed during the 1970s, there are still advocates of separate living arrangements such as 'intentional communities'. These are places set apart from mainstream society, for people with learning disabilities to have a home suited to their own needs. Randell and Cumella (2009) for instance, interviewed people with learning disabilities in a large 'village community' in the UK, and concluded that there were positive outcomes of this type of living option, deriving largely from the opportunity to make friendships with other people with learning disabilities in their own community, and the fact that there was no 'overt subordination' to staff. As is outlined on the Housing Options website (see end of chapter), intentional communities can be supportive and meaningful for some people. They can also offer a safe and caring environment, often in a framework of mutual support and help. 'Disabled people are seen as equal contributors, not passive users of a service' (Housing Options website). However, there are drawbacks too, largely due to the fact that intentional communities can be little more than institutions, which segregate people with learning disabilities from mainstream society. Emerson (2004) used a variety of outcome measures to compare 169 adults with learning disabilities living in 'cluster housing', with over 700 people who lived in dispersed housing in the community. Those in cluster housing had poorer lifestyles, lived with a larger number of people, and suffered restrictions in their everyday activities, when contrasted with those in smaller homes.

Models in which the support is tied to the home

Plans for accommodating people with learning disabilities have traditionally been closely intertwined with the question of appropriate and sufficient support (Simons, 2000). Where a total package of house plus support is offered, that will be referred to in this chapter as 'residential accommodation'. This situation is so 'naturalized' in Learning Disability thinking that the house itself seems to dominate people's lives, with its own rules and requirements.

The concept of 'home' for most people is associated with having one's own private place, somewhere to 'call your own'. For many, it is about choosing and putting your own stamp on the place you live, as it was for Julian Goodwin in the opening story in this book. For most people it implies the notion of stability and belonging. However, these notions of 'home' are often totally left out of the equation for people with learning disabilities, and privacy is very hard to maintain. Other people, especially support workers, are likely to have their own key to the front door, or to intrude without an invitation into people's own private rooms (14 per cent reported this happening in Emerson *et al.*, 2005).

There is usually a distinction made between a 'hostel' and a 'group home'. A hostel can accommodate a large number of people, while a group home is typically an ordinary house, situated on a residential street with neighbours who are not disabled. However, both types of accommodation may:

1. be situated within an ordinary community;
2. offer better opportunities for community-based activities than hospital accommodation;
3. offer higher levels of privacy and choice.

(Emerson *et al.*, 2005: 120–1)

If support is tied to the house itself, then housing outcomes are closely allied to the level of support needs people have. In other words, those with higher support needs (almost by definition) tend to be 'placed' where that support is available, with far less attention paid to the ideas about choice, relationships or privacy. Mansell *et al.* (2002) found that nearly half of residents in homes provided by one national charity had severe behaviour problems, and a significant number had very substantial care or physical needs.

Closure of large institutions has not therefore resulted in the end of institutional life. Aspects of institutional living that still persist in residential homes have been flagged up in robust quantitative studies, and include a life dominated by staff rotas; lack of choice over who you live with (Emerson *et al.*, 2005: 40); fewer opportunities for community contacts and activities (Emerson, 2004); the sense that the house belongs to the staff, not to the people who live there. Because of the far greater number of people with high support needs still moving into residential accommodation in the UK, these factors are far more likely to impinge on their lives than on those with higher-level independence skills.

A systematic review of research evidence was carried out by Hatton and Emerson (1996), and compared the outcomes for people with learning disabilities living in hospitals, hostels, group homes or independent living schemes (see also Emerson 2005: 120–1). Interestingly, there was little hard evidence at that point that the move to 'community based' settings had resulted in improvements in challenging behaviour. There was also little evidence that people with learning disabilities were likely to gain more friends, or to get a paid job, if they moved into 'the community'. However, there was evidence to suggest that people in group homes (i.e. any accommodation 'in the community'):

- had more personal possessions of their own;
- were prescribed less psychoactive medication;
- expressed greater satisfaction about their home;
- enjoyed greater choice of everyday matters;
- had more 'community presence' – i.e. use of community facilities.

In practice, as Hatton and Emerson admit, there is vast variation in the practices of care staff in group homes and hostels, and it is staff support that appears to make the most difference to the lives of people with learning disabilities, which will be considered in more depth in Chapter 9.

Decoupling support from accommodation

Over the past ten or more years in the UK, new ideas have been emerging about offering real housing choices to people with learning disabilities, by changing the way in which the 'bricks and mortar' of accommodation are linked to the support which people with learning disabilities need. Some of these ideas were first articulated by Simons and Ward (1997) and Simons (2000). In models of 'supported living' the notion of where the person should live is separate from the idea of what support they need. This means, in practice, that there is a need: (a) to tackle the issue of how to find houses and flats which people with learning disabilities can rent or part-own; (b) to find out what support will work best for each individual, and ensure that it is provided. The great advantage of this idea is that (in theory) a person could move from one house or flat to another, while taking their own staff with them; alternatively, they could choose to stay where they are living, but to make alterations to the kind of support that is offered.

Supported living, arguably, represents another step along the road to an independent lifestyle, and these options are currently being developed more widely in England and other UK countries. Emerson et al. (2001) in a study of 381 people, with participant interviews as well as quantitative methods, compared small group homes with supported living, in relation to costs, inputs and outcomes. People in supported living were found to have more choice, and a greater number of community based activities. However, they were also more likely to have had their home vandalized, and were considered to be more 'at risk'. Since 2001, supported living has been even more widely applied as a model. However, Fyson et al. (2007) in a qualitative study of four diverse areas in England, found that some supported living services were hardly distinguishable from residential care, and that residents still only had control over small everyday choices in many cases, not over major decisions. This was similar to the picture reported by Coates *et al.* (2004), who reported on a small-scale study of five people with high support needs, and found that contact with other people in the community remained non-existent or superficial for many people living in 'supported living' arrangements. In some cases, residential homes have transformed into supported living arrangements, with very new noticeable changes for residents themselves. Emerson (2005: 123–4) concludes that all these different models of housing can be indistinguishable, and make very little difference in the end to the quality of life for people with learning disabilities.

Despite the wisdom of Emerson's assertion, however, people with learning disabilities still need to have a roof over their heads, and if this is *not* to be simply provided as part of a package of care, then there have to be other options. In the consultation about research priorities carried out by Williams *et al.* (2008b), the priority given to housing was particularly about that issue – how to find actual accommodation. Some of the more innovative thinking in the UK about this question has arisen simply by considering what options anyone in the community has, questioning the assumption that it is always a different, and special, thing for people with learning disabilities to find a home. Having your own tenancy, and simply renting from a private landlord, can be options for some people with learning disabilities. Box 8.3 details some of the ways of becoming an owner of property.

One of the more interesting options over the past decade in the UK has been that of shared ownership, and this will briefly be explored in some more detail, before showcasing one particularly creative way of providing both accommodation and community-based support, via an organization called KeyRing.

Box 8.3   **Housing Options information about becoming a house owner**

- Direct inheritance of family home usually on demise of surviving parent.
- A family purchase a property during their lifetime and then give it to son/ daughter.
- Purchase outright using Support for Mortgage Interest (SMI) up to a maximum loan of £200,000.
- On death of parent or other relative the estate left is sufficient to purchase a suitable property.
- Someone able to earn a reasonable, regular income takes out a mortgage and buys a property in the normal way possibly in conjunction with a gift or inheritance.

In addition to outright ownership someone with a learning disability may become:

- A shared owner.
- A joint owner.

Source: Housing Options Leaflet 14 (see end of chapter)

Creative options for housing

The concept of sharing ownership of a property is very common, among all sectors of society. People will frequently jointly own their property, with a partner, and some may also choose to live with friends or family and buy a house collectively. These options are also open to people with learning disabilities, particularly with the support of their families. However, shared ownership in a more limited sense is taken here to refer to the practice of jointly buying a house, with the support of a Housing Association (King and Abbey, 2010).

In a short article, Workman (2008) describes some of the benefits of shared ownership for people with learning disabilities in Wales, who are likely to gain in self-esteem, and also to have greater flexibility about any potential moves to other areas. The Welsh Assembly government's guidance ('Service Principles and Responses') underlines the right of people with complex needs to live in ordinary housing. The benefits are seen not only in terms of security (since the Housing Association takes on any financial risk) but primarily in terms of greater choice and control for the disabled person. A story is given in Workman's article of someone named 'Jim', in another part of the UK, who has benefited from shared ownership, and the list below summarizes the main points about Jim's story:

1. The Housing Association will support the individual disabled person to work out how much they can afford.
2. Jim himself (with support if he wishes) can choose the location and look out for a property that he likes in the area.
3. Jim still had to pay rent for the share of the house owned by the Housing Association. However, in the UK, it was possible to get housing benefits to help with that.
4. As explained above, it is also possible to get support for paying the mortgage, through Income Support payments.
5. Jim chose to have his support from the same organisation who had provided his previous residential home. However, the support now costs the local authority half the money it previously did.

(based on Workman, 2008)

As Workman points out in her article, capacity to enter into a mortgage agreement could be a problem for some people with learning disabilities. However, the MCA provides for the decision to be taken over by a deputy (either a family/lay deputy, or a corporate deputy), and so this should not stand in the way of making a best interests decision on behalf of Jim or anyone seeking an ordinary life in the community.

However, when people with learning disabilities are housed locally, with personalized arrangements for support, then some commentators have feared that risks will ensue, particularly in relation to financial exploitation (Emerson *et al.* 2009b), lack of ability to maintain the property, and abuse from social care staff employed directly by the person with learning disabilities (Fyson, 2009). While these risks are real, and have to be acknowledged, some creative solutions to housing have attempted to address them through methods which are both about individual choice and also about local communities. One of these is the KeyRing concept (see Resources Section at end of chapter). In brief, the idea is that ordinary housing will be bought up in a small network, with all properties being within walking distance of each other. In one of those houses, there is a support person, who can be called on by those who live in the houses. However, that is only one source of support available to members: the primary resource is seen as mutual support from each other, and indeed from the community around them (Poll, 2007).

Simons (1998) offered an early evaluation of the KeyRing services, and even at that stage, he found significant differences in the approach, as compared with more traditional housing models. For instance, instead of focusing on the 'needs' of vulnerable people in the community, KeyRing has always focused on people's strengths. More recently, the Network has been very interested in finding ways for its members to both draw on local communities, but also to contribute to them as active citizens. An example is given in Poll's chapter, from KeyRing members living in Bristol, the home town for this book:

> With the support of Community Living Volunteers, Network Members have often established good relationships with local police forces and are able to enlist their support on questions of safety. A Community Police Officer in Bristol supported members who were concerned about young people using a derelict flat in their block to take drugs. Members organised a letter from residents in the block and sent it to the Council. A new security system was installed. (Poll, 2007: 61)

Living options for older people with learning disabilities

People with a learning disability in the twenty-first century are increasingly living longer lives (Bigby, 2010; Johnson, 2010). As people become older, there is an urgent need to consider what type of support arrangements, and in fact what type of accommodation, best suits each older person with a learning disability. However, unfortunately, as Thompson (2002) reported, a significant number of these older people are placed in generic older people's homes, where their needs are not well met. Murphy et al. (2009) explored the viewpoints and experiences of older people with a range of disabilities, including a learning disability, and concluded that quality of life depended on a number of factors, in particular focusing on a person's abilities, their access to information and their sense of connection with other people. These types of good practice in support can of course occur in any setting, but all too often are considered unique to services for people with learning disabilities.

A particular issue for some older people with a learning disability is the increased prevalence of Alzheimer's disease particularly among those with Down's syndrome (Strydom et al., 2007; Bland et al., 2003); with a diagnosis of Alzheimer's, the decision then arises about whether people should be supported to stay within their habitual accommodation, or whether they should move to a place where their specific needs could be met more appropriately. Kerr *et al.* (2006) outline the options of ageing in place, in place progression or 'referral out'. Unfortunately, as Watchman (2012) reports from Scotland in a small group of ethnographic cases, people's needs are seldom well met by support services, whatever the type of accommodation chosen. What is needed is more joined-up thinking, and sharing of good support practices, something also emphasized by Bigby and Fyffe (2012) in Australia. Wilkinson and Janicki (2002) suggest some principles of good practice for older people, the first of which relates to person-centred approaches to support: 'an individual's strengths, capabilities, skills and wishes should be the overriding consideration in any decision' (see also Johnson, 2010, for stories told by older people with learning disabilities).

In relation to the mental capacity provisions in England and Wales, research has shown how people are treated, by and large, differently according to their 'dominant' impairment. A typical example of a best interests decision (Williams *et al.*, 2012) was when someone was being discharged from a period of care in an acute hospital. People with dementia in that situation were regularly given time to regain their capacity, and to consider the options open to them, often over a period of several weeks. A particular issue for them was however that 'lack of insight' into their own care needs was sometimes used as a way of claiming that they lacked capacity to decide on where to live. By contrast, younger people with learning disabilities were more likely to be offered good support to take part in decisions about moving home (for instance, by visiting possible places where they may live). However, one older woman with learning disabilities in Williams *et al.* (2012), who had been living in an older people's care home, was considered no longer suitable for this placement once she started developing dementia. People in this situation can be tossed around between the two different 'diagnoses' or dominant identities in their lives. A more joined-up, multi-disciplinary way of working is clearly lacking, but urgently needed, for older people with learning disabilities.

Decision making in practice

Supporting decisions made by people with learning disabilities

In the light of the above considerations about choice, and the limitations placed on people's decisions about moving, this chapter will now consider some recent research about the experiences of people with learning disabilities in making decisions. The two most important factors in moving have been shown to be: (a) who to live with; (b) living in a familiar, local area. For instance, McConkey *et al.* (2003) in Northern Ireland and Gorfin *et al.* (2004) found that the sheer number of co-residents was associated with wanting to move. As in Angela's story (see above), people's experience of home is often coloured by lack of choice relating to those they live with. Further, Noonan-Walsh *et al.* (2001) found in Ireland, when former hospital residents were resettled near their parental home, family members could and did keep in touch on a regular basis. Despite these findings, it is known that in 2006 over 11,000 people with learning disabilities in England were supported in out-of-area placements. This is over one-third (34 per cent) of all people with learning disabilities (Emerson *et al.*, 2008) who are supported in residential care homes and nursing homes, and includes particularly those with higher support needs or challenging behaviour.

How do these decisions affect people with learning disabilities themselves? In a small-scale study, major life decisions in the lives of people with learning disabilities were explored with people in self-advocacy groups (see Chapter 2, pp. 24–5) by Williams *et al.* (2008a). Findings of this study indicated the complexity of most decisions, and the extent to which they took place over time, within multi-party, social interactions. Although the decisions in this study took place before the implementation of the MCA in 2007, nevertheless many of the points of guidance in the MCA Code of Practice proved to be very relevant. The study concluded that those who worked or lived with people with learning disabilities needed to:

- take time to listen and to get to know the preferences of the person they were supporting;
- give good, clear information about available choices;
- provide information in concrete ways, with real-life experience of alternatives;
- make sure that the atmosphere, the place and the time were right for decision making;
- talk with others around the person, as well as with the person themselves.

All this sounds remarkably like good team work. A team approach to decisions is not about making a decision behind someone's back; it is about ensuring that everyone plays their part in finding out information and explaining it in a person-centred way, so that as far as possible, the person with learning disabilities can decide for themselves. Unfortunately, not everyone had this type of experience in deciding where to live. One man in the study told his own story about being moved into a house with a man he did not like, and it was only with the support of his self-advocacy group that he was able to make his voice heard, and to move into more private accommodation.

As personal budgets are put into action in England (see Chapter 2), people with learning disabilities should be able to benefit more from choice and control, by deciding how their own support plan will be formulated. Recent research about support planning has highlighted the importance of person-centred planning (see Chapter 7) where easy, accessible information and continued support from a circle of trusted friends and family can enable a person with learning disabilities to really take a role in constructing their own support plan. Williams and Porter (2011) carried out qualitative research with 80 disabled people, 16 of whom had a learning disability. While all of this group were supported by family members or carers, nevertheless, eight of them had person-centred planning which did enable them to communicate their views and to express their own choices. Of these, three people had made decisions about moving, one from the parental home into a group home, and two from a group home into their own flat. In all these cases, what helped was time to explore the choices, to enable people to get to know the place they may move to, and pictorial means of keeping a record of decisions made.

Best interests decisions about changing accommodation

Despite the overwhelming concern to support people with learning disabilities, as far as possible, to make their own decisions, situations nonetheless arise in which a person lacks capacity to make their own decision. In that case, as mentioned earlier in this chapter, a 'best interests decision' has to be made, and the MCA specifies the way in which this should be done.

One of the important precepts of the MCA is the differentiation of decisions; a person only lacks capacity in relation to a specific decision, a principle which enables people with learning disabilities to be judged capable of some parts of a decision, while needing someone else to take over in other parts. In Williams *et al.* (2012), 385 professionals took part in a large-scale, multi-method study to explore practices in best interests decisions. Interviewees often spoke about the need to define what type of decision the person could manage, and what type they could not. One case was about moving out of a secure ward, into a community setting. The man with learning disabilities in that case was assessed as being able in general to make that decision for himself, in relation to his own independent living. However, he was not able to understand the nature of his own financial commitments and the necessity to budget for bills. Therefore, a best interests decision was made simply in regard to his finances. Once capacity has been assessed, and the decision defined, a best interests process ensues. In major decisions relating to housing, it is possible that a person lacking capacity will have a lasting power of attorney (or 'deputy') appointed, who can act for him/her in legal or financial matters. However, in Williams *et al.* (2012) the authors found that the vast majority of people with learning disabilities had decisions made by a group of professionals, who set up sometimes a string of meetings to seek a consensus about the decision to be made. The MCA guides professionals to make sure that they consult with people close to a person lacking capacity, and find out as much as possible about the person's preferences, past and present. If there is no family member available to consult with, then an independent 'mental capacity advocate' (IMCA) should be appointed, to help with the process. In our research, we found that people with learning disabilities nearly always had a large number of people, family members, staff and others who were involved with any major decision, although the person himself was not often involved directly in the actual best interests meeting. Nevertheless, we heard about many person-centred practices with people with learning disabilities, including the use of Makaton symbols (see Chapter 9) and pictorial systems to assist with communication, and information that included for instance dolls and pictures to try and explain to people what the decision was about. Further, three of the people with learning disabilities in the survey had person-centred plans which allowed others to know in some detail their preferences and needs, and another three had the outcome of the best interests decision recorded for them in an accessible way.

A few cases concerning people with learning disabilities were about risks people posed to themselves. Best interests processes in those cases were very much about protecting people, and ensuring that they had the support they needed to keep safe. One of those cases was explored in some depth, and concerned a man who was putting himself at risk by going out at night and getting involved with drug dealers. The best interests process was about him moving into accommodation where he would have 24-hour support, so that the risks would not occur. Team work and good communication between professionals were vital in that case, and the best interests decision was only raised at the point when nothing else seemed to work. In other words, every attempt was made to ensure that the man with learning disabilities would protect himself from the risks he was taking, in going out at night and meeting with friends who were exploiting him (Williams et al., 2012: Appendix C).

Major best interests decisions were often broken down into sub-decisions. We noted several cases in which the major decision had already been taken, at the point when the person lacking capacity became involved. However, a series of sub-decisions were then explored, and this was the stage when people became more involved. In the interviews, this seemed to be a common pattern with people with learning disabilities. For instance, people who were moving accommodation did not often have a say in whether or not they should move; however, professionals explained how they had involved the person with learning disabilities as much as possible in choosing the place they would go to, selecting furniture, decorations and other matters.

Conclusion: what has the idea of autonomy achieved in relation to housing choices?

The central concept of autonomy has been explored in this chapter from a particular angle, highlighting the legal framework for mental capacity in England and Wales. While 'autonomy' in itself might be a generic policy goal, it has been discussed here in relation to a particular law and professional guidance. As seen in this chapter, the evidence so far suggests that the MCA can in fact make a difference, in providing a clear delineation between supporting decisions and making 'best interests' decisions. However, it also raises some dilemmas about decision making, capacity and best interests, which are relevant for health and social care, and for families and friends of people with learning disabilities. In social care practice in particular, the dilemma faced by staff is the tension between supporting autonomy and protecting their clients by making decisions for them. The notion of best interests itself can be contentious, since it inevitably foregrounds the rights of one individual, sometimes over the rights of others, and in practice there is often a need to balance the needs of family carers with those of a disabled person. Therefore, it is fair to say that the introduction of capacity legislation has served to highlight tensions in the notion of autonomy, which were already in existence, but often ignored.

As seen in this chapter, the decision for people with learning disabilities about where to live is a complex one, and the key to the door may only be found after long deliberation and *joint* work. The 'bricks and mortar' of the house are only one issue; the necessity to have appropriate support is a far greater part of the problem. Therefore, individual autonomy, choice and control are perhaps less important than a collective model of decision making, where people are as involved as much as possible, but where others will also be able to find out information and help them decide. The important practice point here is that people with learning disabilities need to be enabled to get involved with this decision as far as they possibly can, and that full information needs to be given to them – whether they ultimately are assessed as having capacity or lacking capacity. In fact, best interests decisions in the author's research (Williams *et al.*, 2012) were often most successful when they were broken down into different parts. Capacity is perhaps not an 'all or nothing' concept, and as has been seen, people with learning disabilities can sometimes make a decision about where to move, or how to live, without taking full responsibility for every decision in their life. All these aspects of good practice could be more widely disseminated, and could help to keep people with learning disabilities at the centre of decisions in their life.

Another key tension in pursuing autonomy as a goal lies in the overall resource budget that society chooses to allocate to social care or health. As the research summary in this chapter has revealed, however much the MCA may support autonomy, the outcome for individuals depend on local practices, resources and on the availability of personal budget packages which will be able to cover the support needs of *each* person with learning disabilities. Those with the highest support needs are still the most likely to be housed jointly, so that their support can be provided on a cost-effective basis.

Readers may want to reflect on whether life-changing decisions about relocation are made in a 'collective' way in their own lives. It may be that this type of decision looms even larger for people with learning disabilities, since in reality it is not just a decision about choosing a flat or house, but raises issues about how independent the individual can be, what support they will need, whether their family will be nearby, and whether their life will be safe. There is always a wide range of factors to consider, and perhaps the availability of housing itself is not always high on the priority list. For instance, the person called 'Derek' in the BIDS (best interests) research was advised to move into a home where he could have 24-hour support (see Resources, below). The question of where that house would be, what it would look like, whether it would have a garden or a large kitchen, may all be secondary considerations. It is hardly surprising, perhaps, that people with learning disabilities need support to make these complex decisions.

Reflection exercises

1. Think about the principles of the MCA 2005, given in Box 8.1. How are these enacted in practical situations with people with learning disabilities? Work out with others the tensions and difficulties underlying some of the principles, and which would cause the greatest issues in practice.

2. Talk with someone (or a group of people) with learning disabilities, to find out what big decisions they have made in their life. You can help them to map those decisions with pictures, and to find out who else was involved in the decision. Consider what this tells you about individual and collective autonomy.

3. Having a home of one's own feeds into and draws on a person's core identity (Chapter 6) and the right to a private life is also a basic human right (Chapter 3). Building on a discussion about rights, reflect on what systemic changes it would take to give everyone with a learning disability the right to really choose where to live. Consider the roles within a multi-disciplinary team in supporting decisions about housing.

Suggested further resources

1. The Housing Options website has some very useful leaflets and other information about housing for people with learning disabilities:

   www.housingoptions.org.uk

   Other organizations which can help with housing, including shared ownership schemes, are:

   Advance Housing www.advanceuk.org
   Golden Lane www.glh.org.uk
   To find out more about KeyRing, have a look at: www.keyring.org/ Home

2. Resources about the Mental Capacity Act, including information, DVDs and training materials, can be found at:

   www.scie.org.uk/publications/mca/index.asp

   The 'BIDS' report on best interests decisions can be found at:

   www.mhf.org.uk

9 Getting Good Support to Be in Control

Being a personal assistant is a bit like being a shadow in as much as you have to learn to move with your client while not blocking the sun from their face. Your job is not 'to steal their thunder' but rather to allow them to build the confidence that they need to live their lives the way they want to. If that means leaning on you then it should be managed with dignity and with as few people watching as necessary. A colleague of mine calls this 'invisible support'; I call it professional care.

(Clayton, 2006: 138)

The policy theme that has underpinned this book is the mantra of 'choice and control'. Having examined aspects of autonomy in Chapter 8, the current chapter now turns to the element of 'control'. People with learning disabilities regularly say that their lives are controlled by others, but current policy about personalized services aims to turn around the relationship between support staff and those they support. 'We are now the bosses' says a person with learning disabilities in this chapter. A straightforward goal, but it may be trickier to achieve in practice!

Key points summary:

- People with learning disabilities often have other people around them, especially support staff. Their conversations with support staff are a big part of their everyday life.
- Good support means respect. When support staff have too much control over someone, then that makes bad support. This chapter talks about ways of changing the ways support staff treat people with learning disabilities, so that they have a more equal relationship.
- It is important that support workers and carers also have a voice, and that they themselves get good support. People often criticize support staff, but seldom listen to their point of view.
- Successful support is like team work. It is about both partners – the person with learning disabilities and the support worker. It is the job of the support worker to learn carefully what matters for the individual, and to adapt to each person they work for.

Introduction and overview

It is by listening, by interacting and by having conversations that the business of the world gets done, and, in the context of this book, the business of supporting a person with learning disabilities. The experience of everyday life is generally mediated by others. For some people with learning disabilities, that will chiefly involve families; however, as life goes on, people will almost inevitably move beyond the family, and most will live a life in which direct contact with support staff plays a role. The qualities and skills of those support workers are essential – everything else depends on the way support is actually done, and that depends to a large extent on individual personalities:

> Arguably, one of the most powerful actions we can take to improve a person's quality of life is to endeavour to achieve a good match between support worker and client and to ensure that they are compatible. (Harman *et al.*, 2008: 272)

The skills of support workers are therefore a key research priority. Those who were consulted in Williams *et al.* (2008b) felt that existing research had simply not made enough difference in improving standards of support. Since then, there have been renewed scandals in England about abusive practices in the provision of direct care (BBC, 2011), with parallel concerns about the safety of people with learning disabilities who use individual, personalized services and supports. Therefore it is clear that there is still a need to know how to develop better practices in providing the actual services that people need in their everyday lives.

In this chapter, the word 'support worker' will cover everyone who does direct support work, on a regular day-to-day basis, with people with learning disabilities. Support staff can be provided as part of a residential home, as mentioned in Chapter 8. A person living in such a setting therefore may have very little control over who provides their direct support. In other types of living arrangement, the person with learning disabilities can be the tenant, and the support service they access is seen as separate from the house they live in. For instance, supporters may be employed by an organization, but working with one or more people with learning disabilities, as was the case for Julian in the opening story in Chapter 1. With a personal budget (see p. 22), the point is that each disabled person can choose how their support arrangements are realized. In individualised support, the support worker is often called a personal assistant (PA), but whatever the word, this chapter takes the view that what matters is the relationship between supporter and supported. If choice and control are central goals for people with learning disabilities, the choice of one's own support staff must be key to achieving more control in life. Therefore, this chapter will consider choosing and employing one's own staff, and how that can make a difference.

The policy concept on which this chapter will focus is that of 'control', and how that can be achieved through communication practices. Communication is always a two-way event, and much depends on particular conversations, and how they unfold. However, there are tensions in providing support on a basis of equality for people with learning disabilities, many of whom will by definition have significant communication *problems* (e.g. WHO, 2007). Rather than focus on remediation to improve the skills of people with learning disabilities, this chapter is more interested in the consequences of those problems in everyday interaction. The following section of this chapter will consider some of the interactional concepts relating to control, equality and power, before turning to a review of the literature on support staff, while the final parts of the chapter will explore some of the ways in which the concept of sharing control can be applied in practice, by support staff and by people with learning disabilities themselves. 'Extracts' included in this chapter are all transcriptions of real-life interactions, recorded on audio or video camera.

Key policy concept: taking control of one's life

Inequality in communication

Voice of Experience

People often talk to our support workers instead of talking to us, and that makes us cross. People also say 'you're doing well', when you're not. That can sound a bit patronizing.

Source: Members of 'The Voice' group in Williams, 2011: xvii

The foreword to *Valuing People Now* states boldly that:

The strategy focuses on what needs to be done at all levels to deliver the vision of equality and transformed lives for everyone. (DH, 2009a: 2)

As with many of the ideas in this book, a vision of equality is something with which no one would argue. However, in order to achieve it, people with learning disabilities have to regularly take control of their own relationships with those who support them. There are many dilemmas, as this chapter will explore.

Using language in everyday life is one of the central means we all have of achieving our goals with each other. By talking to others, people can praise them, ask for advice, offer them food and a million other things. The study of interaction is therefore not so much interested in the skills and competencies of each communication partner. Analysts are more interested to view talk as action, something that achieves a goal (Wooffitt, 2005: 8).

A particular type of analysis (conversation analysis: CA) is explained more fully in Williams (2011) but is also the basis for much of this chapter. CA explores regular patterns in interactions. For instance, there has been a considerable interest in the way speakers take turns, and in the ways that turns are linked to each other.

When one person asks a question, for example, that gives the other person a 'slot' to answer the question, or to fail to answer. By studying the way these things happen in natural conversations, insights can be gained about talk involving people with learning disabilities. The ordinary, general patterns of talk are still used – but perhaps in some particular ways.

Here is an example of a conversation between a support worker and a person with learning disabilities in Australia:

Extract 9.1

GERALD: So *clears throat* ... *pause* what do you reckon we should *do* with it to thaw it out
WILL: Mm put it in the microwave
GERALD: yep, good thinking
(Rapley, 2004: 179) [transcription conventions removed]

This is a two-way interaction between Will (a person with learning disabilities) and his support worker, Gerald. In some ways, it could be a conversation in any family, where one person is asking another what to do, in order to thaw out some food from the freezer. However, in this particular context, the final comment from Gerald 'Yep, good thinking' gives a clue that perhaps he already knew the best answer. He was simply asking Will a test question, to see if Will could think this out for himself. The support worker formulates the problem, the person with learning disabilities responds and the support worker confirms. This starts to give a feel for the inequality at the heart of Will and Gerald's relationship, and it is one that will probably ring true for many readers who are familiar with conversations involving people with learning disabilities.

Antaki and his colleagues have published a range of papers based on a study of interactions in residential homes and elsewhere, and they confront also the essential inequality at the heart of routine interactions between staff and residents. For instance, they show how staff structure conversations that result in people with learning disabilities appearing incompetent. The following is taken from a discussion between two staff members (Mel and Ann) with residents in a group home:

Extract 9.2

MEL: Right. D'you all know what relationships are?
ANN: Katherine what's a relationship?
KAT: cousins ... niece ... uncle
MEL: *mmm responds to each of these words from Kat*
Tim knows this one don't you Tim?
(Antaki *et al.*, 2007b: 5–6) [simplified and with transcription conventions removed]

Antaki analyses this type of interaction, to show how staff engage in a 'bald operation of power' (Antaki *et al.*, 2007b: 12). That can occur in some very obvious ways; it requires very little analytic skill, for instance, to notice who speaks most, who asks the questions, and how people with learning disabilities can get shut out of conversations. An example is given in Williams (2011: 38) in which a man with learning disabilities is asked 'What about jobs Barry? What other jobs did you have apart from the one you're doing now?' Barry hesitates, and immediately his carers jump in and answer for him. Further, when he is asked for specific information, relating to his previous work experience, his answers are disbelieved and corrected. Inequality can occur when:

1. your chance to speak literally gets usurped by someone else;
2. you do say something, but others do not trust what you say; or
3. you are pushed into speaking up when you do not want to.

If people with learning disabilities are seen as exerting choice and control, with the support worker there simply to listen to what they want, then it would be expected that the disabled person would start up conversations, instruct their support worker, perhaps praise or reprimand when a task is done, and in general set the agenda and tone of the talk, just as anyone would with a paid workman coming into the home. *Inequality* exists when one person has the rights to control the conversation, to set the terms of what is being said and done, and to determine what is correct for the context. Thus inequalities in society can be mirrored and reinforced, each time people talk to each other. For people with learning disabilities, an imbalance of power almost defines their very identity. That is why communication matters, particularly perhaps when one communication partner has extra needs for support.

Equality in communication

Some readers might feel that the type of inequality illustrated above is relatively benign; it certainly does not constitute abuse or neglect, and is a very routine part of the interactions that can engage and develop people's skills. It is not intended here to imply that there are absolute 'right' and 'wrong' ways of interacting with people with learning disabilities. Nevertheless, perhaps by focusing on how equality can be achieved in conversations, the support relationship can be better understood and developed.

A central insight in the analysis of interaction is that people can change the way they talk. Each time two people engage in conversation, they can change the way they think about each other, and the way they make sense of their own relationship:

> Social objects are not given 'in the world' but constructed, negotiated, reformed, fashioned and organised by human beings in their efforts to make sense of happenings in the world. (Sarbin and Kitsuse, 1994: 3)

What then is meant by being in control, through interactions with others, and what would it mean for support staff – who would then have to ensure that the person with learning disabilities can take control? In a study of support skills carried out by the author and co-researchers (Williams *et al.*, 2009a, b, c), the two people with learning disabilities who worked on the project developed five major themes that they felt were essential for good support, on their own terms. The first of these was 'respect'; they sought relationships in which they were respected, treated as adults, and offered advice or guidance only when they wanted it. However, in the twenty or so hours of video footage which we filmed in that study, involving people with learning disabilities and their support workers, there were only two moments at which someone with a learning disability actually told or asked their support worker to do something for them. Equality is, by definition, something to be achieved by *both* parties in an interaction, and the tenets of unequal relationships are deeply embedded in the thinking of people with learning disabilities themselves.

Equal relationships are clearly elusive, and one of the solutions may well be person-centred philosophies. Goodley (1997) has argued that what makes the difference is a true understanding of the social model of disability (see Chapter 2 in this book). In considering support staff practices, then, it is valuable to look beyond the immediate conversation, and explore how communication is situated in the wider beliefs and values of those who occupy that role. The dilemmas occur in actually enacting philosophies of equality in communication practices. Accepting and understanding differences has to be at the centre of support relationships; all too often, support staff are trying to improve or change the person, and perhaps the balance has to swing towards working with an individual on their own terms. Individual control can thus be achievable as a goal, even with those who have the highest level of support needs and communication difficulties, as argued by Nind *et al.* (2010) in the context of disabled children. The key to providing support on a basis of greater equality lies in viewing people with learning disabilities as active agents in their own lives. Before considering how these matters may work out in practice, this chapter now turns to an overview of what is known about support staff practices from the wider research literature.

Research evidence about choice and control

The difference made by personalization

Since direct payments were introduced into UK social services in 1996, research and individual accounts have regularly demonstrated how people with learning disabilities can and do benefit through having a greater sense of choice and control. Participants in a research study in 2000–2 described their lives with direct payments:

Voice of Experience

We are the bosses. We can sit down with the PA and say, now this is what needs to be done. She listens to us.
 My life has changed completely. I used to be in the house all day, looking at the door and the windows. Your mind starts to wander off. I've started now going out to the clubs at night.

Source: Gramlich *et al.*, 2002: 102–3

Those comments were from an inclusive study, in which people with learning disabilities were co-researchers, called *Journey to Independence*. The aim was to explore the support needed by those taking up direct payments, and during the course of *Journey to Independence* project (1999–2002), the numbers of people with learning disabilities in England using direct payments increased from 216 to 900. There was no doubt that, for those able to benefit, direct payments delivered a sense of control and a new-found freedom in managing life in the way people chose, with arguably a 'dramatic and complete reversal of roles' between the person with learning disabilities and their staff (Williams and Holman, 2006: 76). However, the numbers benefiting were still low.

Since that point, the policy of personalization (see Chapter 2, pp. 21–2) has started to transform the way that all social care is delivered in England and Wales, with the advent of personal budgets. Recognizing that not everyone wants to take responsibility for managing a direct payment, the whole purpose of this shift in thinking was to deliver choice and control to *all* those using social care services. Research evidence about the progress of personal budgets for people with learning disabilities has broadly confirmed that:

- People using individual budgets in the pilot scheme were more likely than those in a comparison group to feel they had control over their daily lives, as shown in an influential, multi-methods evaluation (Glendinning *et al.*, 2008: 75).
- Personal budgets have opened up new possibilities for people with learning disabilities to have individual support, on their own terms, in ways that suit them. For instance, in qualitative research, Williams and Porter (2011), people with learning disabilities had one–one supporters who helped them access drama groups or sports centres; they chose group activities to learn about animals or forestry. All of them spoke about or demonstrated their enjoyment, enthusiasm and increased autonomy through that individualized support.
- People with higher support needs, or PMLD (Mansell, 2010) benefit greatly from a personalized approach to their support, delivered through a personal budget and often managed or helped by families.

The problem returned to regularly in research accounts is the fact that many people with learning disabilities cannot manage by themselves all the complexities of running their own support service (Williams and Porter, 2011; Fyson, 2009). Additionally, the Mental Capacity Act 2005 (MCA 2005) (see Chapter 8) has highlighted the fact that some people lack capacity to make decisions relating to their personal budget. New guidance (DH, 2009c) has now introduced the notion of a 'suitable person' so that people lacking capacity can in effect have a third-party payment. Thus much depends on the way in which support and 'brokerage' (see DH, 2008b) is delivered to them, and that is currently being explored by the author in the context of voluntary sector organizations. Findings from Williams and Porter (2011) suggest that it is vital to get the infrastructure right, whereby disabled people's own organizations and other voluntary sector groups can provide the 'enabling' approach necessary for people to exercise choice and control all the way through the personal budget process. Further, there is an urgent need to give better support and back-up to families, who often take on the tasks of managing services for their relative with learning disabilities, particularly those with more complex needs (Coles, ongoing). This situation was also hinted at by proxy respondents in Glendinning *et al.* (2008). One parent in ongoing research recently described a personal budget as a 'poisoned chalice'; it was like a chalice, offering fantastic opportunities to her son with autism and learning disabilities, although it brought with it a massive amount of stress, extra work and commitment into her own life.

Choosing your own staff

The first step in establishing a good support relationship is at the point of choosing staff: who decides how to match support workers to the people they support? Townsley *et al.* (2002) explored staff selection processes in which people with learning disabilities took a key role, and produced and piloted a training pack for staff selection. Since then, despite widespread moves towards personal budgets and direct payments, *Skills for Support* (2005) found that only 31 (52 per cent) of 59 people with learning disabilities who used individualized services felt they had made their own choice for a support worker, although this rose to 87 per cent of those who actually were direct payments employers. Further, it was found that over one-third of those respondents chose a person they knew already. Only eleven people said they had advertised, and eighteen people had taken part in an interview with some support. It would seem then that direct payments do make some difference, albeit with limitations, in enabling people to have a say about *who* supports them.

There are concerns expressed in many quarters about the safety and efficacy of these types of choices (Fyson, 2009) and indeed whether people with learning disabilities would by definition be able to exercise these rights in a neo-liberal climate of personalization (Dowse, 2009). It is therefore essential to have the type of support and help in choosing staff, which will enable people to be 'in control' but with advice and guidance. Support planning in general has thus become a focus of interest in research about personalization in the UK, and Williams and Porter (2011) found that people with learning disabilities benefited from a more continuous, hands-on model of support planning than some of the people with physical impairments. They needed someone who was available for ongoing support to develop their plans, and indeed choose their staff. Where that support was not available, families filled the gap. All six people with learning disabilities in Williams and Porter (2011) who had employed their PAs had effectively chosen them through their parents' recommendation. Equality is a broad term, but a first step is to provide these structural building blocks of personalization, to enable people with learning disabilities themselves to have a voice.

Supporting autonomy

Extract 9.3

FAY: What about some vegetables?
SIMON: *sighs*
FAY: Don't forget those like little frozen packs of vegetables – peas or something
SIMON: I'm not too keen
FAY: not too keen on vegetables?
SIMON: No

(Jepson, 2011: 176) [simplified, and with transcription conventions removed]

A key task for all those who support people with learning disabilities is to support choice. However, in a large sample of 281 people who lived in settings which were explicit about the philosophy of empowerment, Robertson *et al.* (2001b) found paradoxically that people had very little support, even for mundane decisions, and no opportunity to make major life decisions.

The MCA 2005 (see Chapter 8) has further added to the drive to promote choice and autonomy as key goals in support services in general. Jepson (2011) in his Ph.D. thesis cited above used conversation analysis to explore the detail of how this happens in the everyday lives of people with learning disabilities living in residential care homes. By examining the natural interactions that occurred between staff and residents, he showed how choice was foregrounded in the conversations that occurred, whether it was a choice about what food to eat, or a choice about where to go out for a day trip. Support workers regularly used interactional strategies to 'open up' conversations about choice, and to offer different alternatives to people with learning disabilities, so that they were encouraged to think about what they really want. The dilemma, however, occurred when there was a distinction between the decision made and what the support workers knew was the 'good choice'; for instance, in Extract 9.3 a staff member had problems in reconciling the two imperatives (a) to respect a person's choices about food; (b) to persuade that person to eat vegetables. The Mental Capacity Act has a basic principle about the need to honour 'unwise decisions'; yet support workers were continually engaged both in giving choices, but also in moulding and developing people's ability to make the *right* choices. These are difficult issues, which impinge very centrally on what it means to give person-centred support. Other work using conversation analysis has also explored the issue of choice among people with learning disabilities. Jingree *et al.* (2006) for instance showed how power could manifest itself in subtle ways during staff–resident interactions, and in particular via staff failing to acknowledge what residents were saying, while at the same time producing affirmations of service philosophy about choice, through their conversation. Antaki *et al.* (2007a) highlighted a particular feature that staff used, personalizing the choices they offered to people with learning disabilities, by mentioning *people* associated with particular events or activities.

All these studies assume that choice is something that can be offered, by one person to another. The institutional inequality between support workers and people with learning disabilities might only be changed by people with learning disabilities offering choices to their own staff. In one particular case in Williams (2011: 103) that did happen, where a person with learning disabilities set out to offer extra shifts to her personal assistant. However, in general, people with learning disabilities interpreted choices somewhat like tests, and they frequently sought approval that they had made the *correct* choice (Williams, 2011: 92–4). In their training pack, Ponting *et al.* (2010) talked about the notion of control, rather than simply choice. They provided a photo story about the right to change one's mind and 'go with the flow', and they emphasized how they needed the opportunity to choose when and how to have support for their choices. 'Choice and control' are readily available terms for policy, but micro analysis shows that these matters are subtle and difficult to achieve in practice. Clearly, much more evidence is needed about how autonomy can be achieved in everyday support relationships, and about how the principles of the MCA 2005 are enacted in the real lives of people with learning disabilities.

Active support or person-centred approaches?

Despite the advent of personal budgets, Chapter 8 showed that many people with learning disabilities still live in group settings. Since a typical problem in these settings is the passive and disengaged life led by people with learning disabilities (McConkey and Collins, 2010), researchers and trainers in the UK promote a model called 'active support', in which support workers simply engage more directly with the people they are supporting, and enable them to have more involvement in activities generally. The principles of active support are set out in many papers and training materials (Mansell *et al.*, 2002), and are essentially that:

1. Staff provide opportunities for people with learning disabilities to take part in everyday activities – both inside the home and outside.
2. Team work between different support staff helps to ensure that opportunities are offered regularly to the people they support.
3. Just as in good educational models, support workers give assistance as needed, to ensure that people experience success in the activities they carry out.
4. There is a system for recording people's activities, and progress towards taking part and becoming more engaged and active.

Given that active support has an almost inevitable ring of success to it (people who are encouraged to be more active generally do become more engaged), research in this field has turned to finding how support workers can best be trained in these methods. Training courses have frequently been evaluated, and Stancliffe *et al.* (2008) in a special issue of the journal *Intellectual and Developmental Disability* have summarized some of the evidence and developments in this area. It seems that the best way to really change practices, particularly in group settings, is to provide better supervision and direct modelling to staff (Bradshaw *et al.*,

2004). Training courses alone do not make such an impact, since support workers can naturally feel that they do not apply to the people they themselves work with. Support staff in Windley and Chapman (2010) all too often seemed to learn 'by trial and error', and expressed the need for a higher level of on-site supervision, and modelling of good practice.

Despite these positive advocates, 'active support' has its critics. Harman and Sanderson (2008) argued that self-determination is often missing in the active support model; it is the staff who lead by 'filling the available time' for the client. They recommended that person-centred approaches and person-centred plans should be linked explicitly to active support methods, in order to ensure that the activities clients engage in are the ones they themselves want to do. In an exchange of views in the same volume, Jones and Lowe (2008) nevertheless argued that active support is by definition person-centred.

Perhaps an example here would illustrate the issues. If a person with learning disabilities chooses to sit alone in his room, playing computer games, a person-centred approach might involve finding out what interests him about the games, and possibly maximizing on his ability and interests, in order to use them in a different environment such as a workplace. If however the focus is simply on the immediate level of engagement and activity, then the support worker may encourage him away from the computer, and ask him to join other residents in domestic tasks. These are sometimes real dilemmas, since the choices people make in their lives may not always be geared towards increased engagement. As Jones and Lowe (2008) argue, supporting people in a person-centred way can be a key to ensuring that individuals engage with the activities and tasks they themselves wish to. Life should not be a constant lesson about learning independence skills, and the best guide to following a person's own interests and needs is to listen carefully to what they themselves choose.

Providing good support to people who challenge support staff

One of the main priorities for research about direct support to people with learning disabilities has been to examine how best to support those whose behaviour is challenging. Ager and O'May (2001) reviewed over 100 intervention studies, concluding that there was evidence of the effectiveness of behavioural interventions, where support workers analyse the contexts in which certain behaviours occur, and take steps to change the patterns of behaviour. That might involve, for instance, noticing that a person hits out at others when they come too near to him, or appear suddenly in his space, and the intervention might therefore consist both of talking to the person before approaching, as well as praising and developing positive associations, so that the person gradually comes to accept more interaction with others. Grey et al. (2007) found that person-focused training in Positive Behaviour Support resulted in reductions of 30 per cent in the challenging behaviour of residents, which was maintained six months after the intervention. Nevertheless, a review of research in this field (McKenzie, 2011) reports that one of the most frequent ways of tackling challenging behaviour is the use of antipsychotic medication, despite the lack of evidence that these drugs are effective in changing behaviour (Bhaumik *et al.*, 2009: Tyrer *et al.*, 2008). Clearly, there are still some fundamental problems and ignorance about how to support people who challenge the very concept of an equal, social interaction.

A survey of 281 participants carried out by Emerson *et al.* (2001) showed that people with challenging behaviour were far more likely to be living in residential homes than in supported living or other settings; it is therefore residential staff who will encounter most challenges. However, Mansell *et al.* (2002a) found that residential care home staff were least likely to be prepared and were unlikely to have the high levels of skill required. It is also established that moving to smaller, community-based homes can reduce challenging behaviour (McKenzie *et al.*, 2009) and that peripatetic specialist teams can provide useful back-up (Hassiotis *et al.*, 2009). Perhaps therefore one of the clues is to avoid thinking about people with challenging behaviour as so very different in their basic needs. They too will benefit from what we know about establishing good relationships and person-centred approaches to support.

Those who support people who are aggressive face considerable stress in their everyday work; for instance, McKenzie *et al.* (2004), with a sample that consisted of all of those enrolled on a Learning Disability nursing programme, found that 58 per cent of them had been assaulted while working in services. Moreover, support workers may be called upon to physically restrain people with learning disabilities on occasion. Naturally, people with learning disabilities themselves find restraint stressful (Jones and Stenfert-Kroese (2007), Fish and Culshaw (2005) and Hawkins *et al.* (2005) found that staff emotions were high when they were undertaking control and restraint. Support staff can also perceive aggression as an insult to themselves at a personal level (Jahoda and Wanless, 2005), and they may feel 'blamed' for challenging behaviour (Wilcox *et al.*, 2006). Therefore, to improve the type of support given to people with challenging behaviour, there is a need to develop and communicate on a regular basis with support staff, to enable them to understand and think more widely about the causes of the problems they face, and the essential humanity of the people they are supporting. For instance, Tynan and Allen (2002) found that staff who attributed problem behaviour to social explanations were more likely to take some action to prevent problems.

Clearly, despite the continued efforts to establish what works best, there are still dilemmas in providing good support to some individuals with learning disabilities. Indeed, it is in this area that abuse can most easily occur, as mentioned earlier in this chapter. Perhaps one of the basic problems is the separation and 'othering' involved in our habitual approach to people with challenging behaviour. In order to find clues to improving the support relationship, there is a need to consider how the principles of a personalized approach can apply to *all* individuals with learning disabilities.

A reciprocal relationship through non-verbal means

Those people with learning disabilities who find verbal language difficult are often encouraged to use a form of sign language, such as Makaton (see Resources section at end of chapter). Unlike sign languages used in the Deaf community, this is simply a form of visual communication to back up speech and to get messages across. It is often part of an approach called 'total communication', where people are supported through signs, visual and body language, pictures or indeed touch. Each person can develop their own best way to communicate, and it is then important that others learn how to tune in to that individual.

People with profound and multiple learning disabilities rely perhaps the most on satisfying relationships with those who support them, and a detailed, person-centred approach is vital for them. For instance, it is important that staff understand and read the emotions of people with profound disabilities. Support workers themselves often feel that their experience of building relationships is unique, and that it relies entirely on time to get to know the individual. Forster and Iacono (2008) talked with support workers who had all built up a relationship with one woman, called 'Daphena', a woman who communicated primarily with body language. One of the support workers said:

> Communicating with Daphena is about talking to her 'all the time', and believing that she can understand. It is about searching 'what' and 'how' she responds. (Forster and Iacono, 2008: 140)

Shared knowledge of the precise communication strategies of the disabled person can help to create a 'routine' conversation (Mansell, 2010). On the other hand, it has been shown that staff members often make unwarranted assumptions about the intentions of a communication partner with severe communication difficulties (Porter *et al.*, 2001) and that they may then lean towards an activity focus, rather than interpreting communication (Joyce and Shuttleworth, 2001). For instance, it is easier at times to interpret an open-mouthed expression as a 'yes' or an indication of pleasure, so that the planned activity can be carried on. It takes time to realize that it may be a regular way that the person has, to indicate that they feel cold, or perhaps that they are in pain. Clearly, this type of support partnership can work best with some very detailed, structured knowledge about the individual details of how a person communicates. Adams and Oliver (2011) reviewed the research in this field, and concluded that 'multilevel' methods are needed to really understand facial expressions. That can include scanning of eye movements, alongside observations of people's regular reactions, in order to really understand what people are feeling and thinking, when they cannot tell us. A communication passport (Ashcroft, 2002, Millar and Aitken, 2003) can help to explain to new support workers that level of detail, and might be worthwhile for:

- someone whose speech is very hard to understand;
- someone who uses signs, but not necessarily a conventional sign language;
- a person whose main means of communication is through body or facial gestures; or
- people who need particular contexts or circumstances to communicate well (e.g. peace and quiet; standing close to another person; keeping their own distance from others).

Dilemmas in the culture of care

One of the central ethical dilemmas in direct support work with people with learning disabilities, echoed in every account of practice, lies in the necessity to balance protection and risk (Holloway, 2004). White *et al.* (2003) review the literature about abuse, and identify systemic and cultural features of support which can lead to the type of abuse that becomes 'naturalized' and accepted in services. That can include joking, bullying and power issues between staff and people with learning disabilities, issues that are nearly always apparent when institutional abuse comes to light. Unfortunately, official procedures for reporting abuse by staff themselves are not always known or followed (Taylor and Dodd, 2003) and people with learning disabilities themselves tend to be disbelieved (Davies *et al.*, 2005).

It is hard to understand how support relationships with people with learning disabilities can descend into cultures where abuse is simply accepted. People become dehumanized, seen as different, and support workers are driven more by the influence of others they see around them, than by their response to the person with learning disabilities. Even extreme situations of abuse and torture can be overlooked by those whose job it is to inspect for 'quality' care (BBC, 2011), and so it should not surprise us that lesser types of emotional abuse or neglect may not be recognized by those who are perpetrating it.

In general, then, these situations are extreme examples of what is perhaps a general problem of how to translate policy principles such as 'choice and control' or 'equality' into practice. Forbat (2006) for instance, discusses the fact that senior policy executives themselves do not necessarily focus on the key principles of policy, and there is very little guidance about what good practice would look like. Particularly in relation to 'choice and control', there seems to be a fundamental problem which support workers have to work through. While adhering in principle to the rights of people with learning disabilities to make their own decisions, staff also want to make sure people are safe, and that they themselves are not accused of putting people at risk.

In sum, it is known that there are many pitfalls and abysses in the provision of direct support for people with learning disabilities. A good support relationship can be the basis for a good life, as Johnson *et al.* (2010) point out, and we will explore in the following section of this chapter some of the ways that appear to make the difference, in achieving greater 'equality' through person-centred interactions.

Direct support in practice

Opening up and carrying on social conversations

Extract 9.4

FRANK: *taking a cup of coffee from his supporter Adam*
That's just fine cheers. Just how I like it actually

ADAM: Cool. I'm getting better!

FRANK: *laughing* You're not bad at all mate

(Williams, 2011: 82) [transcription conventions removed]

This section turns back to the ideas about communication outlined earlier in the chapter, and explores briefly some of the practice-related understanding that can emerge through studying interactions in fine detail. Most of the examples, including Extract 9.4, can be found on DVD in Ponting *et al.* (2010), which is a resource pack produced with people with learning disabilities, who narrate and present the examples which are given here, showing for instance how Frank and Adam create a friendly, more equal relationship through their jokes and their team work.

Social interaction can only occur between two people if both want to talk. Therefore, the first task for support workers is to ensure there are opportunities to engage a person with learning disabilities in conversation. That can be done in very different ways, resulting in different outcomes. For instance, 'Alice' was a person with learning disabilities, who was filmed sitting at a table in her home, listening to the people around her talk about her future plans for activities (Williams, 2011: 66). Her mother, as well as two support workers went into some detail about these plans, before finally Alice was invited to speak by her mother, with 'Anything you want to say now Alice?' Alice simply said 'no' in a hesitant way, but repeated the 'no' when pressed by one of the support workers. Perhaps she had simply been sidelined in that conversation for too long, and that was the root of the problem, but it should also be noted that the phrase 'Anything you want to say' invites an answer of 'no'. The exact way of phrasing a question can be important.

Later in the same video, Alice responds to an invitation to speak in a quite different way. Here she is walking along the road with Rachel, her second support worker:

Extract 9.5

1. RAC: that's what you did the last time?
2. ALI: yeah
3. RAC: what did you – did you research
4. ALI: I do the *er* … *er er* rugby
   Rachel turns her head to look at Alice, smiles, eyebrows raised
5. RAC: oh? you (want to) look at rugby?
6. ALI: yeah

(Williams, 2011: 67)

Alice has said that she wants to go to the library, in order to use the computer, and Rachel confirms with her at line 1 that this is the same as she has done before. That is a simple yes–no question, and so provides Alice with the chance to just confirm with a 'yeah'. However, Rachel then uses that as an opportunity to follow up with a more specific and demanding question, based on what Alice has said. Essentially the same pattern happens again between lines 4 and 6. This is an easy pattern which seems to work, in terms of bringing Alice into the conversation, and valuing what she has to say. Later on in the video, Rachel and Alice can be seen together in the library, showing through their body language and shared attention how they both have an interest in what is on the computer, which they are accessing together. Once a conversation is started up, then, both partners can contribute, and this can lead to a shared activity – an interest which the support worker and the person with learning disabilities can take part in together.

Shared activities and interests can provide common ground in a relationship, as illustrated in Williams *et al.* (2009b: 611), where a person with learning disabilities has a conversation with his support worker, based on a concert they both went to the previous evening. There is much unspoken detail in this type of conversation, since both parties understand each other and build on what the other has said. That in itself can start to provide the foundation for a more equalized conversation.

It may be considered easier to engage in such 'equal' sounding talk in the context of social chat. What happens during interactions when a support worker has to give guidance or advice? Support workers often have to help manage matters for the person they are supporting, and that can lead to some dominant positioning by support staff. It is certainly not easy to get these things right. In Ponting *et al.* (2010) there are some video examples showing how support workers can loosen the boundaries, sharing more of their own personal lives and encouraging people with learning disabilities to determine the way in which they need to be supported. One man, John, is seen who is writing his own detailed shopping list, in order to budget his money, with guidance from his support worker. There is a to-and-fro between John and his supporter, in which both partners take turns to ask questions, make jokes and enjoy the activity. Significantly, at one point John turns to the camera, and explains that he needs this detailed support 'because of my autism'. That very awareness perhaps gives him some control over the relationship with his support worker, and enables it to develop on a basis of equality.

Supporting people to speak up for themselves

Support workers are not just needed within the home. If one of the support worker's roles is to help people to go out and about, they also need to develop the skills in stepping back, allowing the person with learning disabilities to interact directly with other people. A common and easy scenario is for the support worker to step in, and to speak *for* the person, thus becoming the main recipient in the talk. In the data from Ponting *et al.* (2010), there was more than one occasion on which a passer-by simply greeted the person with learning disabilities directly. Much can be learned from the way in which the conversation then proceeded.

Extract 9.6

1. PASSER-BY: You're not going to watch any rugby then?
2. ALICE: No.

3. SUPPORTER: No not yet. We've just been down the stadium though, to buy her tickets.

(Ponting et al., 2010)

Alice is the same person as in Extract 9.5 above. Here she was walking along with her support worker, when someone she knew stopped to say hello. An understanding of the routine structure and sequencing of turns allows us to see here that the passer-by initiates (what is often called a 'first part') by offering a topic of conversation to Alice: 'You're not going to watch any rugby then?' Alice responds literally to the negative implication of this question, with a 'no'. In some ways, that response is what would be expected. However, there is an additional reason for talking in the street, simply to be sociable, which is perhaps what the passer-by intended. That motive might lie behind what the support worker does, in supplementing Alice's minimal response with 'No not yet. We've just been down the stadium though, to buy her tickets'. The support worker's comment is in third place in the conversational sequence (often called a 'third part') and it does the work of filling out the answer that Alice has already given, thereby keeping the conversation going a little longer, and offering some more information for the passer-by to come back on. However, these matters are subtle. By virtue of filling out Alice's turn in that way, the supporter can easily imply that Alice's original response of 'no' was inadequate, perhaps slightly rude in some way.

These communicative strategies are used intuitively. Another extract in the same data set of videos shows a support worker with 'Archie', someone who does not use words to communicate. The pair have gone together to a youth club, and Archie is talking with his own sign language to his support worker. At one point, Archie uses his familiar gesture for 'tomorrow', and the support worker tells him what he might be doing tomorrow. He then however immediately seizes the occasion to prompt Archie to ask the same question of the youth club leader. The exchange turns out successfully, not only because of the prompt to Archie, but also because the youth club leader has overheard the previous exchange and is therefore more likely to understand the gesture Archie makes, and to respond appropriately. These two extracts are contrasted, in terms of their turn structure, to show how an understanding of CA can help to analyse patterns of talk that are either (a) facilitative; (b) disempowering. At one point, people with learning disabilities can be seen as inadequate, cast as people who may need support to meet and greet a passer-by, while at another point, the three-part structure of a conversation can be turned around to ensure a successful exchange between two people.

It may appear like an ordinary and easy matter, but achieving equality in interactions can require some skill. This is literally about facilitating a person to take control of their life, within the to-and-fro of everyday communication. Many support workers who get to know the person they support, and what matters to them, will do these things naturally. However, they need to learn to step down from positions of power and authority, to listen and follow the lead of the person they are supporting.

Conclusion: are people with learning disabilities more 'in control' of their support relationships?

Support workers are frequently included as research participants, but very seldom as researchers or generators of new knowledge. It is very rare to directly hear the voices of those who carry out support work, although there are some exceptions (Schelly, 2008) and a Ph.D. study about bereavement support which involves support workers as co-researchers (Mason, ongoing). The quotation at the start of this chapter comes from another personal assistant, Clayton (2006), in a volume about direct payments, whose metaphor of 'being a professional shadow' is extremely helpful in understanding the ideal positioning in the support relationship. Direct support relationships are systematically devalued in practice in the UK, and seen as something which can be done by unqualified people or casual labour, and not as part of a professional career. However, establishing a relationship between supporter and disabled person is a delicate, skilled and sensitive task, as this chapter has explored. Until the professional skills of support workers are recognized and nurtured, policies of 'equality' will have a hollow ring. Systemic solutions are needed, not just to train support workers, but to reshape the task of support as a professional career pathway.

This chapter has explored particularly how the concept of equal control relates to communication. It is argued that an analysis and understanding of communication can help to shift and change practice, and that in itself will allow people with learning disabilities to enjoy relationships which are more 'equal'. Their own contribution to those relationships is of course vital, and the subtlety of good support is that it nurtures the person with learning disabilities to become more active in deciding for themselves and taking a full and equal role in social life.

Understanding control and equality also involves a political dimension, and this is reflected in conversation at every level. By analysing the interactions between people, underlying wider societal and policy discourses can be explored. What comes out clearly from the literature and the progress made in research in this area is the value of person-centred approaches to support. Essentially, this means recognizing the fact that everyone is different, and taking the trouble to get to know an individual on his or her own terms. A person-centred plan (see Chapter 7) can help people to understand and appreciate that individuality or 'personhood' of the person with learning disabilities, and to tailor the kind of support that is needed. However, nothing can take the place of the relationship that is at the heart of support work. When it works well, it can become a reciprocal relationship, in which the support worker as well as the person with learning disabilities values what they gain from the work they do. They might find new parts of their own identity, and develop skills and attributes which they did not know they had. Despite this goal, however, it must be remembered that the support relationship is a professional one, and is led by the choices, needs and personality of the person with learning disabilities. It is up to the support worker to adapt.

Having control in one's life is a matter of human rights, as outlined in Chapter 3 of this book. The current chapter has tried to dig down into that abstract notion of control, to examine everyday life, and the way people with learning disabilities are treated in interactions with others. The central tension here lies in the fact that people with learning disabilities do in fact need support to manage their lives, and that can immediately pose challenges to their own independence and equality. It is important therefore to reflect on what it means to 'have control', and how inter-actions can be handled on a basis of equality. It is also important to consider whether changing communication practices alone will be sufficient in bringing about greater control for people with learning disabilities.

Reflection exercises

1. The policy goal of 'choice and control' is easy to remember, but harder to put into practice. In order to apply it to people with learning disabilities, it is important to think about their own contributions and their goals in life. Think of someone you know who has a learning disability, or go and talk with some self-advocates, to find out what their goals are and how they like to be supported.

2. How can support workers treat people with learning disabilities with respect, and what would that imply for their knowledge, skills and understanding? One of the best ways of thinking about your own support skills is to record yourself working with someone with a learning disability. No one is perfect, and it is very hard to avoid being 'bossy', setting the agenda, giving people praise for their achievements and so on. Think about how the conversation could have been shaped differently.

3. In what ways does equality relate to reciprocity and friendliness, when considering support staff relationships with the people they support? Discuss with people with learning disabilities the boundaries of a professional relationship, and the issues about the kind of 'friendly' support they might personally want to enjoy.

Suggested further resources

1. The training pack from Skills for Support is called *Training Your PA* and is available from Pavilion Publishing: www.pavpub.com. It includes a DVD and materials for people with learning disabilities to talk about support skills with their own support worker or PA.

2. For other material and courses for support workers, a good place to start is the British Institute for Learning Disabilities:

   www.bild.org.uk

3. Examples, information, factsheets and guidance about people with learning disabilities taking control of their lives are to be found on the In Control website. It is well worth a visit: www.in-control.org.uk

4. Those who use signs and gestures to communicate often draw on Makaton sign language (www.makaton.org), and there is a range of websites introducing the tools of 'total communication'. One of the most accessible is the Oxford Total Communication website:

   www.oxtc.co.uk

10 Citizenship and Inclusion in Communities

The last policy concept for this book is the overarching concept of citizenship, which brings together many of the previous themes, particularly relating to rights and inclusion. This chapter explores the notion particularly in relation to social inclusion, contributions to communities, and participation in shaping the policies which underpin social and health support.

Key points summary:

- Citizens are people who have rights and responsibilities. Every citizen is part of society. People with learning disabilities are citizens, and can achieve important things that help everyone.
- Unfortunately, the lives of some people with learning disabilities can often seem rather empty and pointless. It is important to change that, and to help people to be good citizens.
- When disabled people talk about independence, they do not mean doing everything alone. People can have support when they need it. It's just the same with being a citizen – people can get support to be a citizen.
- Everyone needs other people, and that is what makes a community. People with learning disabilities can be a strong part of communities.
- Taking part in society means having a voice in politics and government. People with learning disabilities have a voice, through their own self-advocacy movement. They can also work together with other disabled people, so that they become stronger.

Introduction and overview

Despite the UK government's stated commitment to tackle social inequality and exclusion to create an 'opportunity society', people with a learning disability are all too often socially and financially poor – living in the community, but not as part of it. With new policies of community inclusion in England (PSU, 2005; DH, 2005), people with learning disabilities are increasingly receiving individualized services – with the expectation that their activities will be located alongside and

Voice of Experience

I would choose a supporter to take me shopping, and help me do things – go out places. I go out by myself on Saturdays, but on the evenings I don't. I used to have friends where I live in here, but they don't come and see me now like they used to. They used to come in for a cup of tea, but I don't see them now. It's also hard to get a job, there's not much about now, and it's hard for people to get paid work – even if they go to the job centre, or the library, or looking in the newspaper. I can remember when I used to do cleaning, five days a week. That was a paid job, and it used to be good – cleaning an office, and vacuuming. But it's closed down now. In the past there were also day centres, but quite a few of them have closed down now. Mind you, I reckon it's better to have them closed, as people do other things, like going to the drop-in centres. I reckon they prefer that as well. I have friends up at bingo, and I go there every week too.

Source: Kim Norman, in conversation with author, 2012

with other community members and in ordinary community places. UK government policy (DH, 2005: 16, stresses the rights of disabled people to '*contribute fully to (their) communities*'). The same policy document looks towards universal services to prevent social isolation:

> More use of universal services could help people remain better integrated in their communities, prevent social isolation and maintain independence. (DH, 2005: 11)

However, loneliness and isolation can be ever-present dangers for people like Kim, in the comments above. The goal of being part of a community has far wider implications than the saving of societal costs; a fulfilling life for most people revolves around their work role, or their contribution to society, and Kim recognizes how difficult it is for anyone to get paid work.

Disability policies, as Roulstone and Prideaux (2012: 1–20) point out, have traditionally been driven by paternalistic assumptions, whereby disabled people are positioned to be in need of protection and care. In relation specifically to people with learning disabilities, policies are not only about *care*, but also about the hidden motive of *control* (Walmsley, 1999). Recent policy trends have attempted to pull away from paternalism and protection, towards a rights-based model, reflected in the English learning disability strategy (DH, 2001), with its principles of 'rights, independence, choice and inclusion'.

As seen throughout this book, it is well known that the lives of people with learning disabilities differ dramatically from those of others in the community. Policy about inclusion within mainstream services tends to paint a rosy picture of 'community', which in reality may not always exist for a person with learning disabilities. People with learning disabilities in the UK often move exclusively between the community provided by their own family, and the community of a relatively segregated day centre. Some then also move on into other residential services (see Chapter 8) which may provide them with another type of community. As seen in earlier chapters, they frequently live with their families into adulthood (Chapter 5), seldom have a chance to choose who they live with (Chapter 8) and optimistic estimates of those in paid work only amount to some 10–17 per cent. Therefore, compared with other disabled people, their citizenship can appear rather tokenistic.

Nevertheless, people with learning disabilities have started to develop a voice, through their own collective movement for social change, in the UK and at an international level (Dybwad and Bersani, 1996; Goodley, 2000). In fact, UK government policy includes the imperative to listen to those who use services.

> At the same time as giving people greater choice and control over the services they use, we also need to ensure that everyone in society has a voice that is heard. (DH, 2006: 7.4)

In the context of organizations such as People First, the whole notion of participation takes on a new complexion. It is not about providing services to the individual, but about working on a basis of equality with organizations of people who represent others. If disabled people are to be active citizens, then naturally they themselves will be called upon to be partners in creating the plans and policies for the future of welfare and social services (Beresford, 2001; Concannon, 2004). As would be suspected, though, there are some difficult tensions at the heart of collective decision making, which will be unpicked and discussed in this chapter.

The aim here is to explore some aspects of the lives of people with learning disabilities, with a special eye to the notions of equal citizenship, contribution to society and participation in policy making. Some of the models and ideas about 'citizenship' will therefore be considered first, particularly in relation to those who are disadvantaged or socially excluded. We will then pursue research evidence about the daily lives of people with learning disabilities, the extent and rates of employment, community leisure activities and lifelong education. The chapter then returns to the ideas of citizenship, to explore how participation in public policy can be a realizable goal, with collective self-advocacy as the foundation stone, before concluding with some reflections on these terms in relation to the lives of people with learning disabilities.

Key policy concept: citizenship

The nature of citizenship

The idea of citizenship has a long history, often having been synonymous with membership of a society, or even a governmental body. Barbalet (1988) argued that citizenship is a concept that defines who is, and who is not, accepted as a member of a common society. Thus the citizens of Rome were those who could take part in government through a democratic process, and in medieval England citizens were those men of a particular standing, in terms of riches and status, who would have a voice in government. The big question in citizenship theory is therefore about whether it is a conditional, or an unconditional, concept. Does it depend on common humanity (Morris, 2005) or on the particular status, contribution or qualities of the individual?

During the twentieth century, political thinking in the UK swung towards a liberal, social view of citizenship. Marshall's (1950) seminal work helpfully divides the idea of citizenship into three arenas: civil, political and social. Civil rights are the basic freedoms, right to own property and right to justice; political rights are the right to vote, to be part of a political society – enfranchisement. The most influential contribution made by Marshall was in relation to the third arena, that of social rights. Marshall maintains that in a society that is unequal in its distribution of wealth, privilege and status, citizenship cannot be obtained. Further, he makes a distinction between charitable support for those who are less fortunate, and a rights-based approach to universal social equality as a basis for citizenship. Using the example of the Poor Laws in Britain, Marshall argues that it effectively divided those who were citizens (and could contribute) from those who were not. By accepting poor relief, those at the lower margins of society relinquished their chance of being seen as equal:

> The stigma which clung to poor relief expressed the deep feelings of a people who understood that those who accepted relief must cross the road that separated the community of citizens from the outcast company of the destitute (Marshall, 1950: 33)

Marshall coupled these critiques with a vision of a society in which all would have an equal right to a basic income, not dependent on contribution, and where equal 'status' would be conferred on all.

The question for this book has been how far disabled people, and particularly people with learning disabilities, have gained that status, as equal citizens? Since the mid-twentieth century, much has been achieved in the UK and in other societies, towards universal health services, which famously have been 'free at the point of delivery' in the UK, and to a lesser extent, social care services for those who need support in their lives. However, these moves towards social and health care have not always heralded recognition of citizenship. For instance, Oliver (1990) in his analysis of the politics of disablement, shows how the dominant view of disabled people at the time was that of 'individual pathology'. In other words, social care and support were contingent on the problematic nature of individuals. In modern society, as Morris (2005) and other disabled activists have argued (Barnes and Mercer, 2003), disabled people are constructed by social policy as 'objects' of a complex care industry. Further, they have been distanced even further from the attainment of citizenship during the 1980s and 1990s, by a renewed political debate about what it means to be a citizen. Marshall's idealistic vision of social equality has been criticized by neoliberal ideologies for failing to emphasize the *responsibilities* inherent in citizenship.

Various definitions of citizenship have been floated by successive political regimes in England, since Margaret Thatcher's emphasis on contribution and individual achievement. For instance, John Major's conservative government introduced a 'citizens' charter', and Blair's government a test of British citizenship, which would be used to distinguish those who could be counted as citizens and could belong to British society. In order to qualify, a certain level of cultural knowledge had to be shared by all members; that notion of conditional or 'earned' citizenship is an extreme example of shaping individual citizens to the norms of an unchanging, culturally inherited society. Moreover, it could be argued that there is active discrimination here against new arrivals in England, since long-standing citizens do not have to take the test. Indeed, a trial run on the on-line practice test was failed by the current author in 2012. More recent governments have swung increasingly towards the notion of 'active citizenship', in which people have to contribute, not necessarily by financial means, but maybe also by playing active social roles.

Jenny Morris in a very thoughtful essay about citizenship, analyses some of the problems in this conception of active citizenship. As she writes:

> Current debates perhaps focus more on the responsibility to contribute than on the value in itself of people's contribution to the social good – or indeed on the right of people to contribute. (Morris, 2005: 27)

Far from removing disabled people from that obligation, she argues for a swing of the pendulum towards disabled people's own agency, their participation in shaping public policy, and the recognition and inclusion of their contributions in social life. She points out for instance that governmental strategies to promote community volunteering seldom include disabled people, and that funding for disabled people's own organizations is regularly under threat.

The double axis of citizenship, as a status with 'rights and responsibilities' is still very present in English society, and in many other developed societies. In his analysis of disability policy, Drake claims that 'The opposite of citizenship is social exclusion' (1999: 41); in this view, all efforts to dismantle the social barriers that face disabled people are in effect moves towards equal citizenship. Although he acknowledges active citizenship by disabled people, he argues that this should not be a *condition* of attaining citizenship. Disability studies in general has moved broadly within this framework. While claiming the right to have a voice, and to determine policies, disabled people still have to fight back against the notion that they are 'lesser citizens', scroungers on society, or unable to contribute. Morris (2005) argues for a view of citizenship based on the recognition of a common humanity, in which differences are valued. The voice of disabled people, and their contribution, lie at the heart of these models of citizenship, and will be taken up again below.

Citizenship, community and people with learning disabilities

Given the motives and concepts embedded in the discussions of citizenship in the twenty-first century, what place is there for people with learning disabilities? Can they too be equal, both as recipients of social and health care, but also as contributors to society? The theme of 'agency' has been a central one throughout this book, with people's own voices and ideas foregrounded. However, there are some problematic tensions at the heart of this debate for people with learning disabilities.

As seen above, citizenship confers both rights and responsibilities, but it is in effect a status from which disabled people and particularly people with learning disabilities have often unwittingly been excluded (Johnson *et al.*, 2010). The reasons for this are complex, and very much related to the societal view of the identity of 'learning disability'. As Johnson *et al.* (2010) explore, the idea of citizenship is linked with a meaningful life that is all too often premised on the concept of a rational human being. Because people with learning disabilities are commonly believed to lack reason, by the very definition of their impairment, therefore their citizenship is at best conditional:

> The continuing philosophical focus on the importance of reason in defining us as persons and in creating a good life marginalizes people not only social and economically, but also as human beings. (Johnson *et al.*, 2010: 52)

The philosophical notions of shaping one's own life, and of giving value to life through a reasoned awareness and self-determination, are at the heart of what these authors term a 'good life'. The danger, as they outline, is that people with learning disabilities will lead lives that are shaped by others.

The idea of a 'fulfilling life' also raises questions about the meaning of community. English disability policy relies on the idea of a community which could include people with learning disabilities in its activities, social life and public services:

> Services should be person-centred, seamless and proactive. They should support independence, not dependence and allow everyone to enjoy a good quality of life, including the ability to contribute fully to our communities. (DH, 2005: 1.3)

As Duffy puts it: 'citizenship is the word we use to describe what it is to be recognised by other people as an individual who is a full member of the community' (2003: 2). Community is itself a difficult idea to pin down (McConkey, 1998). It can for instance be used to refer to:

- local community – being in the geographical area in which you live;
- communities of people with shared interests and friendship networks; or
- mainstream, as opposed to specialist, services.

In the context of this chapter, the emphasis will be on community as a developing and flexible concept, something that is an action rather than a state of being; people with learning disabilities have several communities, just like everyone else, although some of them may be devalued and even stigmatized. The closure of day centres has been underway in the UK since 1992, when a local authority circular set the direction of day services away from contract work, and towards individually assessed programmes of activities, with greater use of community facilities (Simons and Watson, 2002). As Kim Norman commented in the opening story (above), closure of day centres is probably no bad thing, since most people with learning disabilities have not chosen the 'community' of a day centre. However, alternative communities must then be available, and so more flexible drop-in centres, as Kim said, are a good option. Social isolation is an ever present danger for people with learning disabilities. In this chapter, self-advocacy groups will also be considered as forming communities, where people choose to relate to each other, develop friendships and a collective voice.

Social exclusion and the fight for citizenship

UK government policy since the 1990s has carefully framed disabled people as co-producers, or as autonomous beings who need to shape their own lives. There is also an assumption that 'voices' of people with learning disabilities need to be heard, and that this in itself will help to reverse the social exclusion they face:

> Their voices are rarely heard in public. This needs to change. (DH, 2001: 14)

Nevertheless, the effects of policy have generally been to create disabled people as 'other' (Riggins, 1997: 1–5). Although Riggins claims that 'discourses of otherness are articulated by both dominant majorities and subordinate minorities' (1997: 6), the notion of othering is generally used to describe a process whereby disadvantaged groups of individuals are seen as different, and excluded from the goods of society. As mentioned above, disabled people have long argued that their exclusion is a systemic outcome of the way society is set up (Oliver, 1990). Social exclusion is generally not the result of deliberate action, but is simply the result of the way society is formulated for the advantage of politically powerful groups.

Parallels can be drawn here with other socially excluded groups, such as people from minority ethnic groups, or women. For instance, African-American people in the USA were at one time segregated, given lesser rights to public services, and accepted as second-class citizens. Through raising collective consciousness, however, the movement banded together for change, and achieved a new vision of the status and rights of black people, including predominantly African-Americans. With the election of a black president in 2008, it could be argued that both the rights and responsibilities of citizenship have been endowed on all Americans.

In a similar vein, disabled people in the UK, and elsewhere, formed their own movement (Chapter 2, pp. 12–13 & p. 26), and fought for their rights as equal citizens. The Union of the Physically Impaired against Segregation (UPIAS, 1976) challenged the control and paternalistic care that restricted the liberty of disabled people, arguing for a new way to see disability as arising from social constraints and barriers (Oliver, 1990). Since then, the social model of disability (see p. 12) has been at the very heart of disabled people's own organizations, both in the UK and in other countries (Hayashi and Okuhira, 2008; Singal, 2010). However, can people with learning disabilities have a meaningful place within that picture of liberal citizenship and collective self-determination? As argued by Chappell (2000), and more recently by Dowse (2009), people with learning disabilities have not always been part of pan-disability organizations; their ability to speak up for themselves within the disabled people's movement has sometimes been suspect (Chappell, 2000), and attempts to support people with learning disabilities to develop their own voice are also regularly the object of critique (for example, Redley, 2009).

Nevertheless, in many different countries, people with learning disabilities have banded together and created their own organizations. In some countries these are referred to as self-advocacy groups (see Chapter 2, pp. 24–6) (Sutcliffe and Simons, 1994; Dybwad and Bersani, 1996; Goodley, 2000; Beart et al., 2004), and often have the title 'People First' in the USA, in the UK and in countries as diverse as Germany and Japan.

If full citizenship is something to be fought for, then the collective movement of people with learning disabilities is an important force for change. Although it may not *actively* include the very many different people with learning disabilities in the UK, nevertheless, many would argue that it can still provide a collective and representative voice to argue for citizenship and for rights.

Self-advocacy, participation and contribution by people with learning disabilities

Active citizenship by people with learning disabilities can be viewed at two levels, the individual and the collective. Duffy (2003) for instance, unashamedly focuses on the individuality of citizenship, and urges people themselves (with good support) to activate their own status as citizens, through six 'keys to citizenship'. Duffy's six keys have a strong similarity with the concepts explored in the later chapters of this book, namely 'self-determination, direction (person-centred planning), money, home, support and community life'. Duffy's analysis was strongly linked with the support to be offered through a personal budget, and as such was part of a groundbreaking, practical movement for change in service structures in the UK. It is interesting, moreover, that he frames the whole endeavour as one of the attainment of citizenship. In order to claim their rightful place as fellow citizens, people with learning disabilities and those who support them need to be active in developing *individual* lives. This is a vision in which each person is unique, both in their needs and in their contributions, and Duffy claims that changes at individual level will help to shape and reformulate a more enabling society:

> It is by each of us doing our own bit, by trying to play a full role as a
> citizen, that we will each transform the community into a more
> welcoming place. (2003: 3)

A second type of participation and contribution occurs however through collective movements (see Williams, 2011: Part 2). As seen above, the disabled people's movement is far more than a collection of individuals, but gained its strength from a reformulation of the whole idea of disability. For disabled people generally, the movement for change is almost synonymous with the notion of co-production, and having an active role in shaping public policy (Beresford, 2001).

People with learning disabilities in the UK have also been encouraged to take up active roles in governance and in participation (Concannon, 2004). Both in Australia (Frawley, 2008) and in England (Fyson and Fox, 2008), research has been set up to identify good practice, and to enable understanding of how good part-nership structures work. Since the introduction of *Valuing People* in England (DH, 2001), local social services departments have been required to set up 'partnership boards', which include stakeholders in meetings to discuss learning disability serv-ices. Centrally, this includes people with learning disabilities, but also parents and professionals from other services.

Simply inviting people with learning disabilities to take part in these boards does not, however, ensure an equal voice for all partners. It is notoriously hard to judge mechanisms such as partnership boards on the basis of their achievements – their *product* (SCIE, 2004). It is also hard to distinguish what that product might be, since there has been a lack of clarity about the function and powers of part-nership boards. Concerns have also been expressed about: (a) the process taking over from the product and outcomes of participation (Riddington *et al.*, 2008: 25–6; SCIE, 2004); (b) the role of non-disabled supporters (Redley and Weinberg, 2007); (c) the possibility of meeting overload, where the demands of outside meetings take over from the agenda of people with learning disabilities themselves (Chapman and McNulty, 2004; Fyson *et al.*, 2004); (d) the plausibility of verbal and relatively competent people with learning disabilities representing other, more disabled, individuals (Mencap, 2004; Fyson and Fox, 2008: 35–6); and finally (e) the effectiveness of participation in leading to change (SCIE, 2004). Moreover, there is a notorious gap which often looms between the public persona and status of someone who participates in policy forums, and their own private life (Williams, 2011: 225–6).

Some of these matters will be explored further below. In the meantime, however, it should be acknowledged that tokenism is an ever-present danger in the way in which people with learning disabilities are included within policy forums, and that the idea of 'citizenship' may need to be questioned and rethought in order to really include all people with learning disabilities.

Research evidence about community inclusion

Being part of communities

Research about community presence across the world has often focused on the limited nature of 'community' for people with learning disabilities. For instance, a participatory action research study in New Zealand reports that adults with learning disabilities described their lives as revolving around the safe havens of home and day centre:

Out of cadence with the ordinary social life of the surrounding community and lacking a self-determined compass, the boundaries of participants' community tended to be defined by professional social practices. (Milner and Kelly, 2009: 51)

In 2005, a group of researchers, including carers and people with learning disabilities, set out to map the extent of community-based opportunities for adults with learning disabilities across the UK. The criteria used to measure genuine community opportunities were:

All people, irrespective of the level of support they need, will be –

- undertaking activities that have a purpose;
- in ordinary places, doing things that most members of the community would be doing;
- doing things that are uniquely right for them, with support that meets their individual and specific requirements and overcomes inequalities;
- meeting local people, developing friendships, connections and a sense of belonging.

(Cole *et al.*, 2007: 1)

In other words, this review focused primarily on notions of 'mainstream community', with ordinary places and connections with local people at the heart of activities. This study found evidence that practice outstripped research in matters to do with community inclusion. For instance, people with learning disabilities were increasingly doing things alongside people, for reasons other than having a learning disability, and were supported by a mixture of services during the course of a week, doing a variety of different things. Leisure and sports focused initiatives in particular were opening up opportunities where people *chose* to come together to do things because they shared an interest in what's on offer. Despite the emphasis on mainstream communities, the study also found good examples of social groups,

Box 10.1	The Alumwell project

When neighbourhood housing offices based on local estates in the Walsall district were being disposed of the day services commissioner stepped in and took two over, for free. A partnership has been developed with the Alumwell Residents Trust to develop the building as a community centre for local people. The Trust has used funding from the fair share lottery fund, administered through the Birmingham Foundation, to renovate the building. A local councillor is very involved with the Residents Trust, and a local resident is pushing for it to be really inclusive. There are exciting possibilities for people with learning disabilities to take part in adult education groups, local history societies and to be part of the residents' trust itself.

Source: Cole et al., 2007

where people with learning disabilities got together with each other, gaining support for friendships; some of these took place during the evening as well as the day. Box 10.1 gives an example from Cole *et al.* (2007) of opportunities available at that time, and the types of strategies used to achieve these opportunities.

The goals of community inclusion should be for all. Yet the arguments for community-based services often founder when it comes to those with the highest support needs, namely those with profound and multiple learning disabilities, and those whose behaviour is challenging. It is often assumed that people with the highest levels of support need will still require some specialist solution, such as a day centre, a sensory environment, or a therapeutic centre. In the UK, research on community inclusion for people with high support needs has not been encouraging. Those who are more able seem to have greater opportunities for choice, as measured on a choice scale (Hatton *et al.*, 2004b), and for community presence (Hall and Hewson, 2006). The key factor in influencing community contact for people with learning disabilities appears to be the activity level, commitment and availability of support staff, as evidenced by robust factor analysis (Felce and Emerson, 2001), since without support there are many people who simply do not have the chance to go out, to meet other people, or to be accepted within ordinary activities.

Employment

As argued in this chapter, a citizenship model implies that people with learning disabilities will be active contributors to society, including through paid work. However, the rates of open employment for people with learning disabilities are still very low, even by comparison with other disabled people. For instance, Watson *et al.* (2006a: 28) found that fewer than 10 per cent of people with learning disabilities had regular jobs, compared with 51 per cent of other disabled people, and compared with 81 per cent of non-disabled people. Other research has found that only 6.4 per cent of people with learning disabilities are in any form of paid work (Samuel, 2010). Further, the majority of people with learning disabilities in work were working part time for fewer than 30 hours a week, although slightly more men than women work long hours. The goal of truly open employment is still elusive, and there are many systemic barriers which seem hard to remove. These include the following:

- An inflexible and inaccessible advertising and recruitment process: people with learning disabilities cannot read job adverts, have difficulties with a CV and application, and will also find formal interviews difficult.
- The benefits trap: people who rely on income support, for instance, to supplement their income, will have to relinquish their rights to that benefit if in work. Others will simply not earn enough to pay for the level of their care needs, and will find it hard to make work 'pay' as much as their non-work earnings. For those in residential care, the problems are the most intransigent.
- A job market relying increasingly on high levels of technical skill. The traditional jobs taken up by people with learning disabilities are disappearing fast, for instance – horticulture, car park attendance or simple office work.

While the UK government has pursued a policy of 'welfare to work' for a decade or more, this has had very little effect on people with learning disabilities. Their entitlement to state support for their care has often meant that they are seen as 'incapable of work'. The majority of people with learning disabilities who have moved into open employment have done so with the aid of supported employment services, which are set up specifically for them (by contrast with generally available job centres, or even specialist disability employment advisers) (Wistow and Schneider, 2007; Hunter and Ridley, 2007). The features of successful supported employment have been well documented in (see EUSE in Resources section at end of this chapter) and are given in Box 10.2.

Box 10.2	Features of a successful supported employment service

- A belief in the fact that everyone can work, no matter how 'severe' the disability.
- Work placements organized for clients, in order to establish what people really want from a job.
- Individual profiling available, where the particular skills, talents and preferences of a person are assessed.
- Job matching, where jobs are analysed in detail so that they can be matched to individual job seekers.
- Job coaching, to support the individual worker to obtain work, to access their workplace, and to learn the job.
- Proactive work with local employers, in order to 'sell' people with learning disabilities to them, and to engineer job opportunities.

Although difficult to obtain, open paid employment has been shown to be a cherished goal of many people with learning disabilities. An inclusive research team, set up through a self-advocacy organization in Cornwall, reported in 2012 (Tucker *et al.*, 2012) on their research about different models of supported employment – from the point of view of people with learning disabilities themselves. In addition to the financial incentive of work, there are many documented social benefits (Beyer *et al.*, 2010; Chadsey and Beyer, 2001). People with learning disabilities say that their lives are enriched by work, and that they feel happy that they can achieve something and contribute to society. In other words, they are able through work to be active citizens, rather than passive recipients of care and services.

In order to provide a full range of employment choices that suit people with learning disabilities, it might well be that we have to look beyond the rigid job market as it stands at present. Just as inclusion in education means more than fitting a disabled child into a non-accessible environment, inclusion in employment means paying some attention to shaping and altering the employment market. This can be done, for instance, by creative thinking about partnership work. It is about working with local councillors and the council strategy for all its citizens; developing partnerships with businesses, other providers, churches and faith groups, pressure groups, public facilities, transport services, housing providers, planners. A range of productive partnerships in the employment sector were found in Cole *et al.*'s 2007 research, and these resulted in small work projects, social firms, and the creation of other work opportunities for people with learning disabilities.

Barriers to community inclusion

When people with learning disabilities do engage with their communities, they have increasingly pointed out the problems of bullying and hate crime (Perry, 2004), and in several recent consultations and events they have alerted policy makers to the negative consequences for them. For instance, the English learning disability strategy (DH, 2009a) recognized the importance of hate crime, and planned to take action on the problem. It was also recognized as a need for action research in Williams *et al.* (2008b). To develop truly inclusive communities, issues about attitudes and discrimination will be central problems to tackle. Since then, many local initiatives have been launched to tackle hate crime directly, by involving police forces and community organizations. Mencap launched a three-year national campaign against hate crime in 2011, citing the case of Fiona Pilkington, a mother of someone with learning disabilities who was driven to family suicide through harassment of herself and her daughter. As the Mencap website states: 'Cases like these show that hate crime is still not taken seriously enough by the authorities.'

There are also many other practical problems facing people with learning disabilities in their quest for citizenship in the first decade of the twenty-first century:

- People with learning disabilities themselves do not have knowledge and social skills; support staff are lacking; location of housing can have a negative effect; there may be a lack of community amenities and unhelpful community attitudes (Abbott and McConkey, 2006).
- Transport can be a barrier, as well as the lack of a friend or supporter (Beart, *et al.* 2001).
- There may be insufficient staff in group homes to support people on a 1–1 basis (Reynolds, 2002).

Lack of friends and social networks are also mentioned in many different research studies, although this is perhaps a circular argument – if people do not enjoy full engagement with their communities, then perhaps by definition they are not able to develop friendships (see Chapter 6). The two certainly go hand in hand: personal relationships are the reason for most people wanting to go out and enjoy leisure opportunities, and personal relationships also underpin the value of work and paid employment. Therefore, the matters raised in Chapter 6 will be very pertinent to a full understanding of community inclusion and citizenship.

A final but vital problem for people with learning disabilities lies in their own personal finances. Recent research has emphasized the poverty in which most people with learning disabilities live, and so their ability to get out and have a community life will often be limited by their lack of personal resources. Emerson *et al.* (2005) took the range of items used in the 2000 PSE (poverty and social exclusion) survey to discover how many people could not afford the things in their lives that most adults would want. The results were significant. People with learning disabilities were far more likely not to be able to afford these things than people in general who took part in the PSE survey, which in turn could limit their engagement in community life. Ongoing doctoral work at Norah Fry Research Centre is finding that people who live on the margins of service provision have extensive, interlocking problems, both in 'making ends meet' and in coping with day-to-day life (Tilly, forthcoming).

Citizenship in practice

Nurturing communities

Community is a concept that cannot be taken for granted. Active relationships are required to form communities, as discussed above, and mere geographical co-location does not guarantee that interaction will occur between people with learning disabilities and others. There are two possible responses to that problem, and probably both are needed. Milner and Kelly (2009) in a New Zealand context suggest that it is important not to assume that community is something 'out there' into which people with learning disabilities need to be inserted. Policy about community presence has been blind to the fact that people with learning disabilities create their own communities, through their connections with each other, and within centres, self-advocacy groups and projects. However, a second and complementary response is that communities themselves may need to be nurtured and developed. Clare Wightman is a leading activist in the UK, who has developed a service called 'Grapevine' in Coventry, based on a sound understanding of how to build up networks of sustainable relationships with people with learning disabilities and others:

> The 'crisis' in 'crisis advocacy' is always about isolation, not debt, not harassment from neighbours, not rent arrears. It is isolation, which makes people vulnerable to the crises they present to us. They do not have the network of relationships that might provide aid and support at times of difficulty. The ice under their feet is thin. (Wightman, 2009: 3)

The work carried out by Grapevine was a central part of a project in 2009 by the Foundation for People with Learning Disabilities (Swift and Mattingly, 2009), entitled *A Life in the Community*. One of the main findings from that study was that person-centred planning (see Chapter 7 of this book) was a vital key, so that connections could be made, based on the interests and passions that people with learning disabilities already had. However, active efforts still had to be made to find opportunities to develop those interests, and to involve others in the locality. For instance, one woman with profound disabilities set up a neighbourhood magazine exchange, with the help of her support workers. This enabled all the people in the street to benefit, and to see each other and exchange old magazines – the basis for new networking and friendships.

Individual forms of support are vital to these new ways of working. As was explored briefly in Chapter 2 of this book, the UK government has firmly espoused the agenda of 'personalization', premised on choice and control by disabled people, and often using the tools of individualized funding packages. Glendinning et al. (2008) evaluated the first fourteen pilot sites for individual budgets, and found that for most groups of disabled people, there were considerable gains in quality of life as well as cost–benefits to be obtained, although people with learning disabilities in particular frequently required the support of family and friends in order to benefit. In addition to personal assistants, a new range of professional roles is required, in order to support disabled people to manage their self-assessment, designing their own services, and access community resources. These new roles include those of 'broker', advocate, and peer support worker (DH, 2008b). These may not all be separate professionals, but could be viewed usefully as functions to be fulfilled by different people in each individual's life. For instance, support planning by disabled people's own organizations was found to be very beneficial in Williams and Porter (2011) and an ongoing study by the same authors is focusing particularly on the role of the voluntary sector in helping individuals to work out what they want from their support plan. The skills of community connecting will be vital, in ensuring that people with learning disabilities are enabled to use their individual budget creatively, and to pursue the lifestyle of their own choice. Particularly for those with high support needs, as Swift and Mattingly (2009) found, community connectors need to:

- find out what is available in the local community;
- match activities with individual needs;
- relate well to service providers, club leaders and others who will be able to welcome in the person with learning disabilities; and
- provide the sensitive one–one support which will be necessary for many people to engage with others in their neighbourhood.

Finally, there are many 'specialist assumptions' surrounding people with high support needs, both those with challenging behaviour and people with profound and multiple learning difficulties (PMLD). For instance, it is assumed that some people need a physiotherapist with them, who understands how to move them; it may be assumed that they can only communicate with the help of technology, and that their activities have to include special sensory environments. While all these things may be important, it is possible to break down the chain that leads people with high support needs to be 'contained' in specialist environments. Most of their needs can be met in ordinary locations, with a little creativity. An example from Cole et al. (2007) illustrates this point:

The day service modernisation manager in Nottingham used the PAMIS Changing Places campaign video to help persuade neighbourhood services, chief officers and councillors that work was needed to achieve accessible facilities locally. A working group of Access officers, architects, OTs, physiotherapists, and staff from neighbourhood services created a design and then tried it out using a 'mock-up'. The council has been convinced: the redevelopment of the Market Square in Nottingham will include an adult changing facility, and others are in the pipeline.

Source: Cole *et al.*, 2007

Self-advocacy: active citizenship

The voluntary sector is clearly an important player in the move towards community involvement and in the development of support services at an individual level, reflected in theory within the UK coalition government's 2010 promise to develop the 'Big Society'. As seen above, the notion of 'citizenship' encompasses both social inclusion in communities, but also participation in policy. In this context, how far can people with learning disabilities themselves become active citizens, helping to shape policy and services?

Those belonging to self-advocacy organizations (see Chapter 2, pp. 24–6) have, since DH (2001), had a role in direct representation at local and national level in England, as well as other UK countries. For instance, regional forums representing people with learning disabilities were set up in 2001, electing members to serve on a national forum which reported directly to government ministers. They were able to raise issues such as hate crime, bullying, and also the needs of people with profound learning disabilities, which had a direct influence on policy. For instance, the revised learning disability strategy in 2009 included as priorities some of the matters raised by representatives from the National Forum, including housing and health services.

Despite these seeming successes, direct political representation like this has been critiqued, as tokenistic and as unrepresentative (Redley and Weinberg, 2007), who note how people with learning disabilities taking part in policy forums were in fact speaking up about their own lives, and their personal stories. In formulating policy statements based on their points, however, they stumbled and were not able to operate independently. Instead, they were reliant on non-disabled supporters to speak for them. Redley and Weinberg explain this seeming failure as a direct result of the impairment of learning disability, criticizing the reformist literature which appears to minimize the implications of impairment:

> Our analysis has shown that the PPLD [Parliament for people with learning disabilities], though explicitly designed to honour the liberal democratic principles of political voice and participation, seriously faltered in its efforts to realise these principles in practice. (2007: 783)

In practice, direct democracy of this kind is hard to achieve for anyone, and the lines of communication between 'representatives' and members of an organization are sometimes tenuous. Fyson and Fox (2008: 17–18) refer to this problem as a 'democratic deficit', and attribute it largely to the lack of support to enable consultation to occur. People with learning disabilities are invited to take part in policy forums precisely because of their individual lived experience, and the ability to reflect on that experience has to be fostered and developed. If strong partnerships are based on people taking up different and distinct roles, then the role for people with learning disabilities is a delicate one: they tread the fine path between their personal, lived experience and their public voice as 'representative' for other disabled people. Elsewhere, Williams (2011) has analysed the shift between the personal and the political, the precise ways in which people with learning disabilities can use their individual experiences to make wider, political points (Williams, 2011: ch. 9). Often, this is joint work, supported by others.

Another development springing from *Valuing People* (DH, 2001) in England was the setting up of partnership boards, where local carers, professionals and people with learning disabilities meet together to discuss and plan for local services. Fyson and Fox (2008) in their evaluation of these boards, found some good examples, where the processes of consultation and meetings were altered to suit the needs of people with learning disabilities. For instance, people could co-chair the meetings themselves, ensuring that the agenda was on their terms, and good preparation before the meeting enabled people to think carefully about a particular issue and to speak up meaningfully about it. Nevertheless, for these boards to actually make a difference, it was found to be essential to produce action plans with definite, named responsibility for action. In a review for SCIE (2004), Williams found very similar issues. It was easier for people to focus on getting the *process* of meetings right, but much harder to find examples where anything had *changed* as a result of those meetings.

It may be useful here to consider the various 'ladders of participation' which have been discussed as theoretical frameworks for participation, following Arnstein's (1969) original 'ladder of participation'. The top steps on these ladders generally involve some type of partnership, shared decision making and actual power attributed to those who are 'invited in' on the bottom rungs of the ladder. Although various authors have critiqued the linear nature of these ladders, and some have proposed a more dynamic model, essentially there is a recognition within these models that stakeholders can be invited into partnerships on a step-wise basis. It would seem that all of these models are about developing the power base of the people who are initially the recipients of the services provided by others. In partnerships involving people with learning disabilities, then, it is going to be essential to ensure that a strong self-advocacy or user-led movement exists, which authentically represents the voices of people with learning disabilities. Until that is so, it is hard to conceive of a genuinely equal partnership for change. Australian work on participation with people with learning disabilities, also found this to be a key factor:

> A strong self advocacy movement is a key way to develop the political skills that are fundamental to the meaningful participation of people with intellectual disabilities in government advisory bodies. (Frawley, 2008: 4)

Self-advocacy in government advisory bodies represents the public face of the movement. However, this has to be built on a strong foundation behind the scenes, where people develop their own power. One of the people with learning disabilities who contributed to Williams (2011: 139) spoke about the importance of having their own private space for discussion, without professional managers taking over. He said: 'I'm thinking it's *our* meeting and we run it like what we run it as'.

Creating a knowledge base

Citizenship can be enacted at an individual level, as seen in examples where people with learning disabilities use their personal budgets to connect with local communities; it can also be part of collective action, through self-advocacy and partnership work, arguably developing into political forums for change. However, the most powerful element in the disabled people's movement was the reshaping of thinking about disability, through the proposal of a radical new social model of disability (Thomas, 2004; Oliver, 1990, 2004). How far can people with *learning disabilities* develop their knowledge base, by carrying out research, and establishing their own agenda? Are they de facto included in the knowledge created by other disabled people, or do they have their own issues to contribute? All these questions lie at the heart of debates about emancipatory and participatory research (Oliver, 1992; Barnes, 2003), and the moves towards an 'inclusive research' model, where people with learning disabilities play various roles as initiators, co-researchers, or advisors to research projects (see Marriott and Williams, 2011, for a recent practice-based overview, and also Walmsley and Johnson, 2003; Williams, 1999; Williams *et al.*, 2005). Those who have had experience of working in this way, together with co-researchers with learning disabilities, have often found that their involvement simply makes for better, more insightful research:

> The analysis becomes far stronger and grounded when done with people who identify with the oppressed group. (Williams, 2011: 215)

To what extent, then, can inclusive research be linked with the ideas of active citizenship in this chapter? There are certain well-rehearsed tensions in the notion of people with learning disabilities becoming researchers (Chappell, 2000; Walmsley, 2001), and it remains difficult to get it right – ensuring sufficient support, but maintaining a power balance in favour of people with learning disabilities. In some ways, these practical dilemmas are identical with those faced by people supporting self-advocacy, and indeed by community connectors and support planners at an individual level. If people with learning disabilities need human support to carry out research, does that imply a lack of agency or responsibility on their part? Increasingly, self-advocacy organizations themselves are taking on research projects in the UK, and some examples are given in the 'Resources' section at the end of this chapter. Perhaps citizenship could be reframed within a new model, which does not have to be based on individual, autonomous action, but could be achieved within a collective of joint enterprise, where support is built into the equation. It remains vital to reflect on that support, so that the balance of power is continually questioned and shifted in favour of people with learning disabilities themselves. Yet citizenship and inclusive research go hand in hand and can provide at least one of the platforms for people with learning disabilities to make a difference to policy and practice.

Box 10.4	Inclusive research example

Townson *et al.*, 2007 report on a research study led by the Carlisle People First Research Group. Their research was about advocacy and autism, and people with learning disabilities themselves planned the research and carried it out. For instance, they adapted methods of interviewing, so that participants were more relaxed, and they talked with them both in groups and individually. One of the points which they emphasize in their findings is that, contrary to expectation, people with autism could relate to others in a group advocacy setting – not just at individual level. Their own model of self-advocacy thus inspired them to think of that model as also including people with autism:

> This was very similar to the way a People First self-advocacy group works. The observed group was interested in hearing about People First and started to make suggestions about possible future links.
>
> *Source*: Townson *et al.*, 2007: 532

Conclusion: have ideas about inclusion and citizenship achieved anything?

This chapter has explored some very broad and important themes about inclusion within communities, as well as active participation and citizenship of people with learning disabilities. The fundamental message of the chapter is that fulfilling lives are about contributing, as well as receiving support services, and that as Morris (2005) stated, people with learning disabilities should have a 'right to contribute'. That is part of their citizenship. However, the status of being a citizen should be the starting point, not the end point. The conclusion drawn in this chapter is that it is fundamentally to do with 'being', not 'doing', and people should not be asked to prove that they can accomplish certain tasks in order to earn the status of citizen. If that were the case, some people with learning disabilities would always be excluded. Therefore, we arrive back at Marshall's (1950) conception of social rights as being fundamental to equal citizenship in a society where individual differences are valued.

There are some exciting moves to develop communities, participation and inclusive research, which have been mentioned in this chapter. However, there is also a body of critique about how genuine these initiatives are, and how far they can ever apply to *all* people with learning disabilities. Limitations of cognitive capacity will mean that some people, as Dowse (2009) puts it, will 'never be able to do that'. Perhaps the actual notion of individual citizenship needs to be challenged and rethought, as mentioned above; there may be a place to think about collective citizenship, or even citizenship with support. Just as the disabled people's movement redefined the word 'independence' to encompass the notion of being in control of one's life, with support, so too could citizenship be achieved with some support. The important matter is to ensure that support is delivered in such a way that people with learning disabilities have a clear voice, and self-determination, to develop their own views and to participate fully in the issues they explore. As Townson and her colleagues (2007) in the example above have clearly shown, people with learning disabilities can contribute and support others. Lisa Ponting and Kerrie Ford (2010) similarly developed a training pack based on their research about support skills, and are keen to make a difference to the lives of other disabled people.

It is frequently observed that these empowering ways of working, through inclusive research or in participation forums, rely heavily on verbal and cognitive skills, which single out the few 'able' people with learning disabilities. Nevertheless, people with higher levels of need have been included in several research studies (e.g. Williams, 1999), and can also be supported through creative means to express their own ideas and to 'have a voice' (see Resources section at end of chapter). If it is accepted that people can participate *with* support, then the notion of individual agency may be replaced by supported decision making, whereby people can have a voice within a group of close friends, or can relate to others in communities formulated especially to nurture their own voice.

This chapter therefore also raises questions about what is meant by 'community'. All too often, it is assumed that policies relating to community are about inserting people with learning disabilities into a pre-existing mainstream community from which they have previously been excluded. That type of thinking is very prevalent, not only amongst policy makers, but also amongst people with learning disabilities themselves, who talk about the 'inside' and the 'outside' worlds in their lives. However, people with learning disabilities who have led the way in research projects and self-advocacy act as role models for others, to demonstrate that people with learning disabilities can and do create their own communities. Being a citizen can best be understood as a status based on strength and solidarity with others, and participation in public policy will be more meaningful when it springs from a well-supported collective movement.

Therefore, the final note of this chapter must be to question the separation of 'self-advocacy' from the wider disabled people's movement in the UK. Since the mid-1990s, the relationship between people with learning disabilities and other disabled people has certainly shifted. Townson and her colleagues have published in a leading disability studies journal, *Disability & Society* (Townson *et al.*, 2007), and the Skills for Support research project in Bristol was based within a Centre for Inclusive Living, run by people with physical and sensory impairments. Essentially, the common cause amongst all disabled people is the fact that they identify as an oppressed minority, excluded in various distinct ways from a society that is formulated without any of their needs in mind. That oppression can include the social positioning which disabled people face on a day-to-day basis, as well as the attitudes that exclude them from mainstream communities. The social model of disability may have been critiqued and reshaped in recent years (Thomas, 2004; Goodley, 2011), but essentially it is a tool for change, as Oliver (2004) has eloquently explained in 'If I had a hammer'. People with learning disabilities can also take up that hammer, giving them more strength to have a voice in their own lives, and in disability policy.

Reflection exercises

1. 'Community' in policy and in personal experience can mean very different things. Thinking first about your own personal experiences of 'community', do these opportunities exist for people with learning disabilities? What types of support could be envisaged to nurture inclusive communities for people with learning disabilities?

2. Think broadly about what citizenship means. You may want to go to try out the UK practice citizenship test, and see how you do! You can find it at:

    www.ukcitizenshiptest.co.uk

    Discuss other meanings of citizenship, and consider whether the term represents something that is achievable for people with learning disabilities.

3. A fulfilling life can look very different for each individual. Much depends on a person's individual goals and sense of identity. Talk with some people with learning disabilities known to you, and find out what aspects of achievement are important for them in their own lives.

4. In practice, supporting community inclusion can involve some very specific information and skills from a range of practitioners, both inside and outside learning disability services. Work out a community map of who may be involved with a particular individual, by thinking creatively 'outside the box'.

Suggested further resources

1. The report Life in the Community is available from the Foundation for People with Learning Disabilities at:

    www.learningdisabilities.org.uk/publications

2. At the same website, you will also find Claire Wightman's account of the work of Grapevine in building real community connections for young people with learning disabilities in Coventry. www.learningdisabilities.org.uk/publications/connecting-people

3. The Mencap campaign against hate crime can be found at:

   www.mencap.org.uk/news/article/hate-crime-campaign-launch-during-learning-disability-week

4. Several self-advocacy organizations in the UK and elsewhere have their own websites. See for instance, Dorset People First (2010) Citizenship Project. www.dorsetpeoplefirst.co.uk/library/citizenship.pdf

5. Cornwall People First was mentioned in this chapter, as they have carried out inclusive research about employment:

   www.cornwallpeoplefirst.com/projects/work_in_progress

   Supported employment across Europe is developed and promoted by the European Union of Supported Employment (see their website: www.euse.org/ where you can find very useful 'how to' guides and a supported employment toolkit).

6. Finally, a recent project by Mencap produced a resource to help people with profound and multiple learning disabilities have a voice, and there are some wonderful videos to view and discuss at: www.mencap.org.uk/involveMe

11 Promises, Practices and Real Lives

Overview of the book: how have the 'big ideas' in policy fared?

This is not a substantive 'final chapter', and does not aim to repeat the concluding remarks about citizenship on preceding pages. Instead, the story of policy and practice for people with learning disabilities is an ongoing one, and so the end point of this book is better framed as a snapshot, glancing back at some of the issues raised by various chapters and looking forwards to the future.

What has policy ever done for people with learning disabilities?

Each chapter of this book has highlighted a particular policy concept, and attempted to follow it through via research evidence, into practice. In doing so, inevitably, there is some analysis and critique of the concept itself. However, on the whole this book has adopted a positive stance, as outlined in Chapter 1, with the aim of exploring as far as possible what each idea has to offer people with learning disabilities themselves. The gaps between policy and practice are often bemoaned, as they were in the research priorities work carried out by the authors in 2008 (Williams *et al.*, 2008b); it is instructive therefore to review the extent to which the various policy concepts in this book have influenced practices, and what factors might underpin that link. Moreover, it could be argued that the choice of one particular policy term for each chapter is somewhat arbitrary. There are deep links between all the concepts, and it can easily be seen how one theme is only meaningful by reference to others.

A good example of that interlinking is the first concept explored, that of human rights. Essentially, the notion of human rights underpins all the chapters, not simply the issues to do with health care in Chapter 3. However, if the right to life is considered fundamental, then equal access to health care is clearly an essential starting point (Emerson and Baines, 2010: Mencap, 2007). In order to improve health services for people with learning disabilities, the idea of 'human rights' has to be operationalized. Therefore, Chapter 3 also draws on the fundamental notion of inclusion, whereby the institutions of society (in this case, health care institutions) are reshaped in order to respect and support *all* individuals (Robertson *et al.*, 2010). The same arguments put forward about inclusion in Chapter 4 could apply equally to health care, as they do to education. Further, the ideas of autonomy, choice and better communication practices are also very central to the arguments about health (DH, 2009a). Where improvements in access to health care have been observed, for instance through the implementation of annual health checks for people with learning disabilities, then they tend to draw on all the concepts highlighted in this book. A system that honours the different needs of all its citizens is one which is truly universal, and essentially is linked with the notion of citizenship explored in Chapter 10. Many other examples could be given of the interdependence of the various ideas in this book, and their translation into practice. Readers may wish to trace some of the practice developments back to the ideas presented across the book, rather than simply to the theme highlighted in each chapter.

This perceived interdependence of policy ideas raises the question: why do words matter? Can policy rhetoric affect the lives of people with learning disabilities, and why do we need so many new headline words, to change and improve the life chances of any individual in society? In exploring the concepts throughout this book, it has become apparent that the real purpose for banner headlines is to provoke reflection, and in fact to challenge previous conceptions of learning disability. The social model itself is a prime example of that type of challenge, since by positing an alternative, medical model, it set up the idea of disability as social oppression by contrast to prevailing attitudes. In doing that, Oliver (1990) and his colleagues used a new type of language about disabled people, in order to critique and unpick what was wrong about current disability policy. Similarly, the notions of 'inclusion' and of 'choice and control' can be used as challenges, when applied either to people with learning disabilities themselves or to their families. In Chapter 4, it was argued that inclusion in education should be seen as a right for all children (Barton, 2003), and not as an option, where disabled children are inserted into a system which does not really encompass their needs. Translating this idea into practice results in whole-school systemic changes towards individual planning for *all* children. The inclusion of children with learning difficulties can therefore be seen potentially to benefit all students.

Nowhere is the notion of challenge more salient than in Chapter 6, with its focus on identity and relationships. The idea of people with learning disabilities as having emotions, being sexually active, and as choosing the option of parenthood, are all challenging to prevailing ideas (Abbott and Howarth, 2002). In exploring 'identity' as a key theme, we are uncovering and questioning the assumptions that lie beneath existing practices, such as the Irish Sexual Offences Act 1993 (see Chapter 6, pp. 104–5), and the lack of support for parents with learning disabilities. The Working Together with Parents network in the UK (Tarleton, 2009) is a prime example of policy challenge being linked with practical change, so that attitudes can be shifted towards greater acceptance and positive support for good parenting.

Practices linked to policies

The policy concepts in Chapters 7 and 8 are slightly different, since they are linked with actual tools for change. In Chapter 7, the tool is that of person-centred planning, which has arguably had a major influence on shifting the life outcomes of people with learning disabilities (Robertson *et al.*, 2005). Effectively, it offers a bridge between the idea of individual autonomy and social support for people's lives. Good person–centred planning (Sanderson, 2000) continues to focus maximally on what the individual person *wants,* by understanding the unique nature of each personality and each person's dreams in life. It is a great example of the effective translation of policy into practice, through a practical toolbox of strategies that can be adapted by people in different circumstances. In a different way, the notion of autonomy is put under the spotlight in Chapter 8 within the context of the Mental Capacity Act 2005 in England and Wales (Williams *et al.*, 2012). A legal framework can perhaps have the greatest effect in achieving change, since it has 'teeth'; if a person's wishes are not taken into account and supported, if they do not receive a fair and balanced assessment of capacity, or if their best interests are not properly and transparently decided on, then cases can be challenged in the courts. It is important that research continues to monitor the outcomes and effects, both of person–centred planning and of the Mental Capacity Act.

The focus on interaction in Chapter 9 raises the question of who is in control. Again, like other concepts, this is an idea that is built on the analysis of *inequalities,* in the ways in which people with learning disabilities are routinely treated by those around them. The analysis of 'naturally occurring data' (Antaki *et al.*, 2007a, b) is as close as we can get to what actually happens in the everyday lives of people with learning disabilities, and by using this type of analysis to inform training and reflection, support practices can be directly improved (Williams, 2011; Ponting *et al.*, 2010). The aspects of policy that have proved perhaps the most valuable are those that can be operationalized into practical tools, such as person–centred planning in Chapter 7, or specific initiatives such as the parents' network in Chapter 6. However, it is the systemic change towards personal budgets that has the potential to deliver the greatest shifts in people's lives, if it is backed up with sufficient resources, support and facilitation. That was evident in Chapter 9, in relation to support staff practices, but also in Chapter 10, with the links with citizenship and community involvement.

The impact of policy on the real lives of people with learning disabilities

All the policy terms in the current book can and are used to promote debate, and allow the wider public to engage in more critical thinking about the role of people with learning disabilities in our society. Citizenship, as argued at the end of Chapter 10, is a key example of such an overarching, public debate. By reflecting on the difference between 'conditional' and 'unconditional' citizenship, the rights and responsibilities of people with learning disabilities can be promoted. Active citizenship is highlighted through the examples in the 'Living in the Community' project (Swift and Mattingly, 2009) as it also is through participation work and self-advocacy. Inclusive research, as demonstrated in this book, can be powerful and challenging too, but needs to be considered alongside a range of different types of evidence. Lisa Ponting, from the Skills for Support team, was involved in research, and looked back at the project on a video made in 2008.

Voice of Experience

This research gives us power, and that's how we get listened to. I remember coming for an interview here, and People First helped me to do that. It was great to get the job. Before I got this job, I didn't know about research. I did in a way, because I was doing things with People First, but I'd never actually gone out and carried out what I'd learnt with People First … Research is thinking about people's lives, and what they do with it. And also, how they get their support. Because remember, we were looking at the support. People have their own views on their own subject. And what we tried to do was to listen to them, and to take their views, as they'd take our views. But we hope that this will make a difference. The thing is, what has this project done for disabled people? What we have done will make a benefit for other disabled people.

Source: Lisa Ponting, July 2008

By contrast with the mid-twentieth century, some people with learning disabilities undoubtedly now have lives that have benefited in some ways from ideas about equality and citizenship, as Lisa Ponting expresses above. Moreover, this is not just about being 'done to': disabled people can and do provide expert support to each other. This book has demonstrated by reviewing a range of different types of research in each chapter how certain policy themes, such as inclusion and autonomy, have in fact delivered gains for people with learning disabilities.

However, despite the efforts of Lisa, and other active citizens with learning disabilities, the very real conditions of social exclusion, poverty, lack of employment and lack of choice in housing are all still very evident in the lives of people with learning disabilities, as robust, often large-scale, studies have demonstrated. Despite legal frameworks and public debates about citizenship, inclusion or partnership, people with learning disabilities still face many barriers in society. Moreover, there are large numbers of people with more complex learning disabilities, who are not so able to speak for themselves and are dependent on people who know them well to interpret their preferences. The extent to which they benefit from inclusive policies is less immediately evident, and qualitative research struggles to find new ways to observe and understand this group. Therefore things are never straightforward and simple and it remains vital to keep questioning the effectiveness of policy rhetoric. Perhaps the question now becomes: apart from personal budgets, annual health checks, inclusion for some children in education, early support partnerships, and an increasing number of person-centred plans – what *has* policy ever done for us? The next section will consider where the threats to progress may lie.

General and current threats to people with learning disabilities

As outlined above, this book makes no apology for pursuing essentially progressive and empowering notions of citizenship in relation to policy and practice for people with learning disabilities. However, it has also unearthed some of the tensions and competing forces, which often stand in the way of achieving the 'big ideas' of policy. Essentially, these can be divided into three areas: (a) ideas about what it means to have a 'learning disability'; (b) the need for services to meet different goals which sometimes conflict with each other; (c) arguments about overall allocation of society's resources.

What does it mean to have a 'learning disability'?

A frequent reason for disregarding idealistic notions about citizenship or autonomy relates to the definition of 'learning disability', which implies a difficulty in managing life, in communicating, making decisions and acting as an autonomous human being. There is a continuous tension therefore between protection of people who are seen as vulnerable, and their empowerment through progressive policies and practices, which was outlined in Chapter 2 (p. 16; see also Dowse, 2009; Fyson, 2008). The question for readers to resolve is how that balance between autonomy and protection can be achieved. In each chapter, the need to provide good support has been posited alongside the notion of independence, so that successful outcomes for people with learning disabilities are based on that sensitive balance. For instance, in Chapter 9, achieving more equal interactions with support staff is set alongside the need for support staff to protect, guide and advise people with learning disabilities. That is precisely why the task is so difficult, and why the theme of 'advice' was pursued by Lisa Ponting and Kerrie Ford (Ponting et al., 2010). These self-advocates concluded that the important thing for them was to get good guidance, on their own terms, when they needed it. They thus positioned themselves as autonomous, thinking beings, who could be in control through a meta-level of awareness of their position in life.

Understandably, others with learning disabilities, including those with PMLD, may find that level of control and awareness more difficult to achieve. Nevertheless, this book has explored several ways in which they too can remain central to the decisions in their lives – with the support of families (Chapter 5), through person-centred planning (Chapter 7) and with the implementation of best-interests decisions under the Mental Capacity Act (Chapter 8). An inclusive society is one in which the different needs of all its members are accepted within a common framework of citizenship. By focusing on that notion of supported citizenship, each individual's needs for safeguarding as well as empowerment can be encompassed. The danger in some of the current analyses of policy is that the progressive concepts of rights and empowerment can easily be discarded, in favour of more traditional, safe or protective mechanisms of care. However, it is all too clear that the paternalistic social care response of 'specialist services' can backfire and turn into abusive, even torturing, environments for people with learning disabilities (BBC News, 2011). Exploring creative, personalized support does not mean leaving people open to unnecessary risks, and the major challenge today in many countries is to find ways to ensure people really are safe, on their own terms and with their own individual supports.

Competing goals in health and support services

The policy concepts explored in this book can all be seen as ideas that set the direction of travel for support services, or for society at large. However, the evidence in each chapter has shown how difficult it is to measure through systematic research evidence real achievements in travelling towards those goals. Perhaps one of the fundamental reasons is that the organizations and institutions of society are pulled in many different directions, and often therefore fall back on what is termed the 'logic of practice' (Bourdieu, 1990). At an individual level, people do what they do because they are part of an organizational culture which dominates their actions.

Examples of these dilemmas can be found throughout this book. For instance, in Chapter 4 the notion of 'inclusion' in the education system has to be set against the achievement of targets, and the league tables by which English schools are judged. In order to survive and be seen as successful, head teachers therefore have to ensure that curriculum targets and examination results are not compromised. When faced with a pupil who needs extra support, a teacher may therefore feel frustrated that their time is unduly occupied by one student, at the expense of others. Similarly, in Chapter 9 a support worker who spends time on a daily basis with people with learning disabilities may have to help people who challenge through their behaviour; she or he may also have to protect people from the risks posed by their own choices, including for instance their choices relating to food or exercise. Therefore, there are competing tensions here between supporting autonomy and what is known as the 'duty of care'. What often happens is that the support worker will fall back on what works in particular circumstances, and develop practices that seem right within the team or the context in which they are working. The relationship between support services and families (Chapter 5) masks the extreme tension between blame and partnership; as seen in that chapter, family problems can easily be tipped into 'problem families'.

Some of these dilemmas raise the question of power, and the unequal distribution of power between the different players involved in supporting people with learning disabilities. Research that links the 'micro' with macro issues such as power remains very relevant, as reviewed in Chapter 9 and elsewhere in this book. Although the mantra of 'choice and control' puts the person with learning disabilities themselves in the centre (Chapter 7), they are surrounded by a matrix of other powerful individuals – family members, support workers, social services staff, doctors or psychologists. Power can be vested in individuals who have particular forms of expertise, as well as a hold on the purse strings of public money. Therefore, parents in Chapter 5 for instance can feel that they are being asked to work in partnership, but on the terms of the professionals' agenda. The Mental Capacity Act (Chapter 8) may be intended as a personalized piece of legislation, but it can also be seen to privilege the expertise and power of the person who leads a best interests decision. More open reflection and communication about some of these issues would certainly help, but there are no easy answers. To change the power balance and ensure more equal opportunities, it is important that all parties approach each other with the rights of the person with learning disabilities centre stage.

Allocation of money from the public purse

Personalization however is not necessarily the answer to everything. Personalized services themselves have been critiqued for relying on a general motive to save money from the public purse. The current crisis in social care across Europe is fuelled by public fears about growing numbers of older people who will require care from the state in the coming years. In systems where the social care budget is situated close to the individual, the bureaucratic infrastructure is dismantled, and money more effectively spent on direct needs and outcomes. A programme of research studies for the School for Social Care Research in England is currently reporting on how personalization is succeeding or struggling, across England and Wales. Dismantling of unnecessary bureaucracy may be beneficial, but losing trusted group activities or services may be counter-productive. At a deeper level, the notion of individual responsibility for one's own support services can be critiqued as being symptomatic of the dismantling of the very welfare state itself. Personalization can thus be seen both as a win–win situation for state and service user, but also as a threat. What may lie beneath these dilemmas is the difficulty of shifting power from the state systems to disabled people and their allies, with good partnership work and support to enable all those concerned to play their role to full effect.

Policy in the UK thus currently reflects some contradictions in society. Perhaps the thinnest policy rhetoric of all is that of the 'Big Society', in which the government claims to promote community actions and self-help, among all sectors of society. At the same time, all these initiatives are currently suffering from a reduction in actual budgets, and long-term insecurity. Voluntary and user-led organizations that have previously played important roles in participation and co-production of social supports are increasingly faced with cuts, while individuals managing personal budgets are also struggling to make ends meet. Strong personalized policies require commitment in terms of funding.

In this climate, people with learning disabilities face many threats. Not least, their need for public funding can be used as a spark to ignite harassment and abuse from others in society, who themselves feel undervalued or underprivileged. Disability hate crime in the UK in general is on the increase, and the notion of undeserving disabled people who are 'benefit scroungers' is also applied to some people with learning disabilities. In this climate, the future may appear bleak. However, it is all the more necessary to remain value driven, and to ensure that the gains made in recent years in policy and practice are maintained. A body of good practice exists in the UK, Australia, Canada and elsewhere to promote person-centred approaches, choice and personalization. Essentially, the notion of citizenship lies at the heart of all these. With the countries of Europe and America generally facing similar financial crises, globalization of policy and practice can therefore provide an opportunity for people with learning disabilities. Solutions found in one context may well apply to another, and international links between practitioners and people with learning disabilities themselves can lead to reflection on shared values and human rights debates.

Disability studies and self-advocacy

Voice of Experience

Self-advocacy means speaking up for yourself. if you don't speak up for yourself, you bottle things up for yourself. We've got to feel – we've got to be personal in our lives as well, to speak out ... you've got to really pour it out.

Source: Self-advocates' discussion, Williams, 2002: ch. 4

Leading self-advocates in the above discussion were reflecting on what the term 'self-advocacy' meant for them at the turn of the millennium in the UK. Since then, the movement has developed and organizations grown in coherence, and in strength, across the UK and in many other countries, including Japan, Germany, Canada and North Europe. At the same time, during the first decade of the twenty-first century, policy in England and Wales has made some decisive moves to include people with learning disabilities as direct participants. No longer should they have a voice that is 'silenced' and be represented only by others who have their interests at heart. Therefore, every important policy forum now needs to question whether or not people with learning disabilities have a voice to express and reflect on their lives. Academic research projects, local partnership boards, government reports – all have to demonstrate that they have fully taken into account the viewpoints, as well as the needs, of those with learning disabilities.

In the debates about disability policy, the lead 'user' voices are still those of disabled people who do not have cognitive impairments. That could be seen as inevitable, since academic analysis of policy requires a high level of cognitive ability, which by definition is going to be hard for people with learning disabilities to achieve without support. However, some of the leading exponents in disability studies in the UK have a background in working with people with learning disabilities (Goodley, 2011, for instance) and regularly include their voices and engage with them in debate. That is what the current book has also tried to do. Similarly, in the field of personalization, it is the practices pioneered by people with learning disabilities and their families that have often led the way in England. For instance, person-centred planning tools can have far wider application than simply in the field of Learning Disability.

The disabled people's movement has to remain open to those without academic credentials. The challenge for the movement is to really find ways of including the viewpoints and experiences of people with learning disabilities, on a basis of equality and respect. The challenge for people with learning disabilities is to find ways to make their own voices heard, within and alongside those who experience disabling barriers in different ways. Many of the difficulties faced by disabled people in Western societies in the twenty-first century will be similar for all groups, whatever the impairment, although some will have a particular resonance for particular groups. The debates about policy and practice however need to be conducted in an inclusive spirit, where everyone has a voice, and it is to be hoped that the current book will contribute to those more open discussions, involving all disabled people.

References

Abbott, D. and Howarth, J. (2002) *Secret Loves: Hidden Lives*. Bristol: Policy Press.

Abbott, L., McConkey, R. and Dobbins, M. (2011) 'Key players in inclusion: are we meeting the professional needs of learning support assistants for pupils with complex needs?, *European Journal of Special Needs Education*,26(2) 215–31.

Abbott, S. and McConkey, R. (2006) 'The barriers to social inclusion as perceived by people with intellectual disabilities', *Journal of Intellectual Disabilities*, 10: 275–87.

Abraham, C., Gregory, N., Wolf, L. and Pemberton, R. (2002) 'Self-esteem, stigma and community participation amongst people with learning difficulties living in the community', *Journal of Community and Applied Social Psychology*, 12: 430–43.

Adams, D. and Oliver, C. (2011) 'The expression and assessment of emotions and internal states in individuals with severe or profound intellectual disabilities', *Clinical Psychology Review*, 31: 293–306.

Adams, L., Beadle-Brown, J. and Mansell, J. (2006) 'Individual planning: an exploration of the link between quality of plan and quality of life', *British Journal of Learning Disabilities*, 34: 68–76.

Adler, G. (2010) 'Driving decision-making in older adults with dementia', *Dementia*, 9(1): 45–60.

Ager, A. and O'May, F. (2001) 'Issues in the definition and implementation of "best practice" for staff delivery of interventions for challenging behaviour', *Journal of Intellectual and Developmental Disability*, 26(3): 243–56.

Ainscow, M. (1999) *Understanding the Development of Inclusive Schools*, London: Farmer Press.

Alborz, A., Glendinning, C. and McNally, R. (2005) 'Access to health care for people with learning disabilities in the UK: mapping the issues and reviewing the evidence', *Journal of Health Services Research and Policy*, 10: 173–82.

Antaki, C., Finlay, W. M. L., Jingree, T. and Walton, C. (2007b) '"The staff are your friends": conflicts between institutional discourse and practice', *British Journal of Social Psychology*, 46: 1–18.

Antaki, C., Walton, C. and Finlay, W. (2007) 'How proposing an activity to a person with an intellectual disability can imply a limited identity', *Discourse and Society*, 18(4): 393–410.

Antaki, C. and Widdicombe, S. (eds) (1998) *Identities in Talk*, London: Sage.

Armstrong, D. (2002) 'The politics of self-advocacy and people with learning difficulties', *Policy and Politics*, 30(3): 333–45.

Armstrong, F. and Barton, L. (2008) 'Policy, experience and change and the challenge of inclusive education: the case of England', in L. Barton and F. Armstrong (eds), *Policy, Experience and Change: Cross Cultural Reflections on Inclusive Education*, Dordrecht: Springer Science, 1–18.

Arnstein, S. (1969) 'A ladder of citizen participation in the USA', *Journal of American Institute of Planners*, 35(4): 216–24.

Arthur, A. (2003) 'The emotional lives of people with learning disability', *British Journal of Learning Disabilities*, 31: 25–30.

Ashcroft, E. (2002) 'Communication passports: towards person-centred planning', *Living Well*, 2(4) 11–13.

Atherton, H. and Crickmore, D. (eds) (2011) *Learning Disabilities: Towards Inclusion*, London: Churchill Livingstone.

Atkinson, D., Jackson, M. and Walmsley, J. (eds) (1997) *Forgotten Lives: Exploring the History of Learning Disability*, Kidderminster: BILD Publications.

Atkinson, D. and Walmsley, J. (1999) 'Using biographical approaches with people with learning difficulties', *Disability and Society*, 14(2), 203–16.

Azmi, S., Hatton, C., Emerson, E. and Caine, A. (1997) 'Listening to adolescents and adults with disabilities from South Asian communities', *Journal of Applied Research in Intellectual Disabilities*, 10: 250–63.

Barbalet, J. (1988) *Citizenship: Rights, Struggle and Class Inequality*, Milton Keynes: Open University Press.

Barnes, C. (2003) 'What a difference a decade makes: reflections on doing "emancipatory" disability research', *Disability and Society*, 18(1): 3–17.

Barnes, C. and Mercer, G. (eds) (2003) *Disability Policy and Practice: Applying the Social Model of Disability*, Leeds: Disability Press.

Barnes, C. and Mercer, G. (2006) *Independent Futures: Creating User-Led Disability Services in a Disabling Society*, Bristol: Policy Press.

Barton, L. (2003) 'The Politics of Education for All', in M. Nind, J. Rix, K. Sheehy and K. Simmons (eds), *Inclusive Education: Diverse Perspectives*, London: David Fulton Publishers and Open University Press.

Baum, S. and Burns J. (2007) 'Mothers with learning disabilities: experiences and meanings of losing custody of their children', *Learning Disability Review*, 12: 3–14.

Baxter, H. Lowe, K. Houston, H. Jones, G. Felce and Kerr, M. (2006) 'Previously unidentified morbidity in patients with intellectual disability', *British Journal of General Practice*, 56: 93–8.

BBC News (2006) 'Sick baby's family thanks judge', http://news.bbc.co.uk/1/hi/health/4808442.stm

BBC News (2009) 'Baby in right-to-life battle dies', http://news.bbc.co.uk/1/hi/uk/7956845.stm

BBC News (2011) 'Government condemns "shocking" Winterbourne View abuse', www.bbc.co.uk/news/uk-13617196

Beart, S., Hardy, G. and Buchan, L. (2004) 'Changing selves: a grounded theory account of belonging to a self-advocacy group for people with intellectual disabilities', *Journal of Applied Research in Intellectual Disabilities*

Beart, S., Hardy, G. and Buchan, L. (2005) 'How people with intellectual disabilities view their social identity: a review of the literature', *British Journal of Learning Disabilities*, 18: 47–56.

Beart, S., Hawkins, D. Stenfert, Kroese, B. Smithson, P. and Tolosa, I. (2001) 'Barriers to accessing leisure opportunities for people with learning disabilities', *British Journal of Learning Disabilities* 29: 133–8.

Beresford, P. (2001) 'Service users, social policy and the future of welfare', *Critical Social Policy*, 21(4): 494–512.

Beyer, S. Brown, T., Akandi, R. and Rapley, M. (2010) 'A comparison of quality of life outcomes for people with intellectual disabilities in supported employment day services and employment enterprises', *Journal of Applied Research in Intellectual Disabilities*, 23(3): 290–5.

Beyer, S., Grove, B. *et al.* (2004) *Working Lives: The Role of Day Centres in Supporting People with Learning Disabilities into Employment*, London: Department for Work and Pensions, Report 203.

Bhaumik, S., Watson, J., Barrett, M. *et al.* (2011) 'Transition for teenagers with intellectual disability: carers' perspectives', *Journal of Policy and Practice in Intellectual Disabilities*, 8(1): 53–61.

Bhaumik, S., Watson, J. M. and Devapriam, L. *et al.* (2009) 'Aggressive challenging behaviour in adults with intellectual disability following community resettlement', *Journal of Intellectual Disability Research*, 53(3): 298–302.

Bigby, C. (1997) 'When parents relinquish care: the informal support networks of older people with intellectual disability', *Journal of Applied Intellectual Disability Research*, 10(4): 333–4.

Bigby, C. (2000) 'Life without parents: Experiences of older women with intellectual disabilities', in R. Traustadottir and K. Johnson (eds), *Women with Intellectual Disabilities: Finding a Place in the World*, London: Jessica Kingsley, 69–86.

Bigby, C. (2010) 'Growing old', in G. Grant, P. Goward, M. Richardson *et al.* (eds), *Learning Disability: A Life Cycle Approach to Valuing People*, Milton Keynes: Open University Press, 663–84.

Bigby, C., and Fyffe. C. (2012) *Services and Families Working Together to Support Adults with Intellectual Disability. Proceedings of the Sixth Roundtable on Intellectual Disability Policy*, Bundoora: La Trobe University.

Black-Hawkins, K. (2010) 'The framework for participation: a research tool for exploring the relationship between achievement and inclusion in schools', *International Journal of Research and Method in Education*, 33(1): 21–40.

Blair, J. (2009) 'Parents as allies', *Learning Disability Today*, 9(4): 22–4.

Bland, R., Hutchinson, N., Oakes, P. and Yates, C. (2003) 'Double jeopardy? Needs and services for older people who have learning disabilities', *Journal of Learning Disabilities*, 7: 323–44.

Bollands, R. and Jones, A. (2002) 'Improving care for people with learning disabilities', *Nursing Times*, 98: 38–9.

Booth T., Booth, W. and McConnell, D. (2005) 'The prevalence and outcomes of care proceedings involving parents with learning difficulties in the family courts', *Journal of Applied Research in Intellectual Disabilities*, 18: 7–17.

Bostrom, P., Broberg, M. and Hwang, P. (2010) 'Parents' descriptions and experiences of young children recently diagnosed with intellectual disability', *Child: Care, Health and Development*, 36(1): 93–100.

Bourdieu, P. (1990) *The Logic of Practice*, Oxford: Polity Press.

Bradshaw, J. McGill, P. Stretton, R. *et al.* (2004) 'Implementation and evaluation of active support', *Journal of Applied Research in Intellectual Disabilities*, 17: 139–48.

Brandon, T. and Charlton, J. (2011) 'The lessons learned from developing an inclusive learning and teaching community of practice', *International Journal of Inclusive Education*, 15(1): 165–78.

Brechin, A. (1999) 'Understanding of learning disability', in J. Swain and S. French (eds), *Therapy and Learning Difficulties: Advocacy, Participation and Partnership*, Oxford: Butterworth–Heinemann, 58–71.

Brewster, J. and Ramcharan, P. (2005) 'Enabling and supporting person-centred approaches', in G. Grant, P. Goward, M. Richardson and P. Ramcharan (eds), *Learning Disability: A Life Cycle Approach to Valuing People*, Buckingham: Open University Press, 491–514.

Bridgen, P. and Lewis, J. (1999) *Elderly People and the Boundary between Health and Social Care 1946–91: Whose responsibility?*, London: Nuffield Trust.

British Institute of Human Rights (BIHR) (2006) *Your Human Rights: A Guide for Disabled People*, bigwww.bihr.org.uk/resources/guides

Brookes, M. and Alberman, E. (1996) 'Early mortality and morbidity in children with Down's syndrome diagnosed in two regional health authorities in 1988', *Journal of Medical Screening*, 3: 7–11.

Brown, M. and MacArthur, J. (2006) 'A new research agenda: improving health care in general hospitals', *Journal of Clinical Nursing*, 15: 1362–70.

Brown, H. and Smith, H. (1992) *Normalisation: A Reader for the Nineties*, London: Tavistock/Routledge.

Brown, R. *et al.* (2011) 'Family life and the impact of previous and present residential and day care support for children with major cognitive and behavioural challenges: a dilemma for services and policy', *Journal of Intellectual Disability Research*, 55(9), 904–17.

Bruner, J. (1996) *The Culture of Education*, Cambridge, MA: Harvard University Press.

Buckner, L. and Yeandle, S. (2007) *Valuing Carers: Calculating the Value of Unpaid Care*, London: Carers UK.

Burton-Smith, R. (2009) 'Quality of life of Australian family carers: implications for research, policy and practice', *Journal of Policy and Practice in Intellectual Disabilities*, 6(3): 189–98.

Cambridge, P. and Carnaby, S. (eds) (2005) *Person-Centred Planning and Care Management with People with Learning Disabilities*, London: Jessica Kingsley.

Campbell, J. and Oliver, M. (1996) *Disability Politics: Understanding Our Past, Changing Our Future*, London: Routledge.

Caples, M. and Sweeney, J. (2011) 'Quality of life: a survey of parents of children/adults with an intellectual disability who are availing of respite care', *British Journal of Learning Disabilities*, 39(1): 64–72.

Carmichael, F., Hulme, C. *et al.* (2008) 'Work–life imbalance: informal care and paid employment in the UK', *Feminist Economics*, 14(2): 3.

Carnaby, S. (2004) *People with Profound and Multiple Learning Disabilities: A Review of Research about Their Lives*, London: Mencap.

Carr, S. (2010) *Personalisation: A Rough Guide*, Adult Services Report 20, London: Social Care Institute for Excellence.

Carson, I. and Docherty, D. (2002) 'Friendships, relationships and sexuality', in D. Race (ed.), *Learning Disability: A Social Approach*, London: Routledge, 39–153.

Cassidy, G., Martin, D. M., Martin, G. H. B. and Roy, A. (2002) 'Health checks for people with learning disabilities: community learning disability teams working with general practitioners and primary health care teams', *Journal of Learning Disabilities*, 6: 123–36.

Caton, S. and Kagnan, C. (2007) 'Comparing transition expectations of young people with moderate learning disabilities with other vulnerable youth and with their non-disabled counterparts', *Disability and Society*, 22(5): 473–88.

Chadsey, J. and Beyer, S. (2001) 'Social relationships in the workplace', *Mental Retardation and Developmental Disabilities*, 7: 128–33.

Chapman, R. and McNulty, N. (2004) 'Building bridges? The role of research support in self-advocacy', *British Journal of Learning Disabilities*, 32: 77–85.

Chappell, A. (2000) 'Emergence of participatory methodology in learning difficulty research: understanding the context', *British Journal of Learning Disabilities*, 28: 38–43.

Clark, D., Garland, R. and Williams, V. (2005) 'Promoting empowerment: your life can change if you want it to', in P. Cambridge and S. Carnaby (eds), *Person Centred Planning and Care Management for People with Learning Disabilities*, London: Jessica Kingsley, 67–83.

Clarke, S., Garner, S. and Gilmour, R. (2007) 'Home, identity and community cohesion', in M. Wetherell, M. Lafleche and R. Berkeley (eds), *Identity, Ethnic Diversity and Community Cohesion*, London: Sage, 87–101.

Clayton, A. (2006) 'The professional shadow: a personal assistant's account', in J. Leece and J. Bornat (eds), *Developments in Direct Payments*, Bristol: Policy Press, 137–8.

Clegg, J., Murphy, E., Almack, K. and Harvey, A. (2008) 'Tensions around inclusion: reframing the moral horizon', *Journal of Applied Research in Intellectual Disabilities*, 21: 81–94.

Clegg, S. and McNulty, K. (2002) 'Partnership working in delivering social inclusion: organisational and gender dynamics', *Education Policy*, 17(5): 587–601.

Coates, S., Barna, S. and Walz, L. (2004) 'A life more ordinary', *Community Care*, 1530: 34–5.

Cole, A. and Williams, V. *et al.* (2007) 'Having a good day? Report of a survey of community-based day opportunities for adults with learning disabilities', London: SCIE.

Cole, B. (2005) '"Good faith and effort?" Perspectives on educational inclusion', *Disability and Society*, 20(3): 331–44.

Concannon, L. (2005) *Planning for Life: Involving Adults with Learning Disabilities in Service Planning*, Abingdon: Routledge.

Contardi, A., Lastella, A., Vulterini, P. *et al.* (2006) *I am, ergo I love*, European Union: Socrates Grundtvig Program.

Cook, C., Williams, K., Guerra, N. and Sadek, S. (2010) 'Predictors of bullying and victimization in childhood and adolescence: a meta-analytic investigation', *School Psychology Quarterly*, 25(2): 65–83.

Cornwall People First (2010) Work in Progress, www.cornwallpeoplefirst.com/projects/work_in_progress

Coyle, K. and Maloney, K. (1999) 'The introduction of person-centred planning in an Irish agency for people with intellectual disabilities: an introductory study', *Journal of Vocational Rehabilitation*, 12: 175–80.

Cumella S. and Martin, D. (2004) 'Secondary healthcare and learning disability: results of consensus development conferences', *Journal of Learning Disabilities*, 8: 30–40.

Danforth, S. (2000) 'What can the field of developmental disabilities learn from Michel Foucault?', *Mental Retardation*, 38(4): 364–9.

Davies, R., Northway, R., Jenkins, R. and Mansell, I. (2005) 'Abuse of people with learning disabilities: everyone's responsibility', *Llais*, 75: 17–20.

Davies, C. and Jenkins, R. (1997) '"She has different fits to me": how people with learning difficulties see themselves', *Disability and Society*, 12(1): 95–109.

Davies, J. and Morgan, H. (2010) 'What kind of future for young people with Down's syndrome? The views and aspirations of young people and families', *Tizard Learning Disability Review*, 15(4): 22–9.

Davies, J., Burke, C. and Mattingly, M. (2011) *We Can Dream: Ways of Planning for the Future for Young People with Autistic Spectrum Disorders*, London: Foundation for People with Learning Disabilities, www.learningdisabilities.org.uk

Davies, M. and Beamish, W. (2009) 'Transitions from school for young adults with ID: parental perspectives on "life as an adjustment"', *Journal of Intellectual and Developmental Disability*, 34(3): 248–57.

Dawkins, B. (2008) Memorandum on behalf of the PMLD Network by Beverley Dawkins (Mencap) to the Joint Committee on Human Rights, www.publications.parliament.uk/pa/jt200708/jtselect/jtrights/40/40we67.htm

Dawkins, B. (2009) 'Valuing Tom: will valuing people now change the lives of people with profound and multiple learning disabilities?', *Tizard Learning Disability Review*, 14(4): 3–12.

DCSF (2007a) *Aiming High for Disabled Children: Better Support for Families*, London: TSO.

DCSF (2007b) *The Children's Plan: Building Brighter Futures*, London: TSO.

DCSF (2007c) *Background Information: People You May Meet*, London: TSO.

DCSF (2009) *The Lamb Enquiry: Special Educational Needs and Parental Confidence*, London: TSO.

DCSF (2011) *Support and Aspiration: A New Approach to Special Educational Needs and Disability*, London: TSO.

De Fina, A., Schiffrin, D. and Bamberg, M. (2006) 'Introduction', in A. De Fina *et al.* (eds), *Discourse and Identity: Studies in Interactional Sociolinguistics, 23*, Cambridge: Cambridge University Press, 1–23.

Della Sala, S. and Anderson, M. (eds) (2012) *Neuroscience in Education: The Good, the Bad and the Ugly*, Oxford: Oxford University Press.

Department for Constitutional Affairs (2007) *Mental Capacity Act 2005 Code of Practice*, London: TSO.

Department for Work and Pensions (2006) *Improving Work Opportunities for People with a Learning*

Disability: Report of a Working Group on Learning Disabilities and Employment: A Report to Ministers and the Learning Disability Task Force, London: TSO.

DfES (2001a) *Special Educational Needs: Code of Practice*, Ref: DfES/581/2001, London: TSO.

DfES (2001b) *Schools Achieving Success*, Government White Paper, London: TSO.

DfES (2003) *Every Child Matters*, Government Green Paper, London: TSO.

DH (1996) Community Care (Direct Payments Act) 1996: Elizabeth 11. Chapter 30. London: TSO.

DH (2001) *Valuing People: A New Strategy for Learning Disability for the 21st Century*, London: TSO.

DH (2003a) *Making Things Happen: First Annual Report of the Learning Disability Task Force*, London: TSO.

DH (2003b) *Fair Access to Care: Guidance on Eligibility Criteria for Adult Social Care*, London: TSO.

DH (2005) *Independence, Wellbeing and Choice: Our Vision for the Future of Social Care for Adults in England*, London: TSO.

DH (2006) *Our Health, Our Care, Our Say*, London: TSO.

DH (2008a) *Putting People First*, London: TSO.

DH (2008b) *Good Practice in Support, Planning and Brokerage*, London: TSO.

DH (2008c) *Local Authority Circular LAC Transforming Adult Social Care*, London: TSO.

DH (2009a) *Valuing People Now*, London: TSO.

DH (2009b) *Health Action Planning and Health Facilitation for People with a Learning Disability – Good Practice Guidance*, London: TSO.

DH (2009c) *A Summary of Changes to Direct Payments*, London: TSO.

DH (2010a) *Prioritising Need in the Context of Putting People First: A Whole System Approach to Eligibility for Social Care: Guidance on Eligibility Criteria for Adult Social Care*, London: TSO.

DH (2010b) *Personalisation through Person-centred Planning*, London: TSO.

Diez, A. (2010) 'School memories of young people with disabilities: an analysis of barriers and aids to inclusion', *Disability and Society*, 25(2): 163–76.

Doughty, H. and Allan, J. (2008) 'Social capital and the evaluation of inclusiveness in Scottish further education colleges', *Journal of Further and Higher Education*, 32(3): 275–84

Dowling, S., Manthorpe, J., Cowley, S. (2007) 'Working on person-centred planning: from amber to green light?', *Journal of Intellectual Disabilities*, 11(1): 65–82.

Dowse, L. (2009) '"Some people are never going to be able to do that": challenges for people with intellectual disability in the 21st century', *Disability and Society*, 24(5): 571–84.

Dowson, S. and Greig, R. (2009) 'The emergence of the independent support broker role', *Journal of Integrated Care*, 17(4): 22–30.

Drake, R. (1999) *Understanding Disability Policies*, Basingstoke: Macmillan Press.

Duffy, S. (2003) *Keys to Citizenship: A Guide to Getting Good Support Services for People with Learning Difficulties*, Birkenhead: Paradigm.

Duggan, L. and Brylewski, J. (1999) 'Effectiveness of antipsychotic medication in people with intellectual disability and schizophrenia: a systematic view', *Journal of Intellectual Disability Research*, 43: 94–105.

Dybwad, G. and Bersani, H. (eds) (1996) *New Voices: Self-Advocacy by People with Learning Disabilities*, Cambridge, MA: Brookline.

Dyson, A. and Gallannaugh, F. (2008) 'Disproportionality in special needs education in England', *Journal of Special Education*, 42(1): 36–46.

Eayrs, C., Ellis, N. and Jones, R. (1993) 'Which label? An investigation into the effects of terminology on public perceptions of and attitudes towards people with learning difficulties', *Disability, Handicap and Society*, 8(2): 117–27.

Elliott, J., Hatton, C. and Emerson, E. (2003) 'The health of people with learning disabilities in the UK: evidence and implications for the NHS', *Journal of Integrated Care*, 11: 9–17.

Ells, L. J., Lang, R., Shield, J. P. H. *et al.* (2006) 'Obesity and disability: a short review', *Obesity Reviews*, 7: 341–5.

Elvish, J., Hames, A., English, S. and Wills, C. (2006) 'Parent with learning disabilities: an audit of referrals made to a learning disability team', *Learning Disability Review*, 11: 26–33.

Emerson, E. (1995) *Challenging Behaviour: Analysis and Intervention in People with Learning Disabilities*, Cambridge: Cambridge University Press.

Emerson, E. (2004) 'Cluster housing for adults with intellectual disabilities', *Journal of Intellectual and Developmental Disability*, 29: 187–97.

Emerson, E. (2005) 'Models of service delivery', in G. Grant, P. Goward, M. Richardson and P. Ramcharan (eds), *Learning Disability: A Life Cycle Approach to Valuing People*, Buckingham: Open University Press, 108–27.

Emerson, E. and Baines, S. (2010) *Health Inequalities and People with Learning Disabilities in the UK: 2010*, Lancaster: Learning Disabilities Observatory.

Emerson, E., Barrett, S., Bell, C. *et al.* (1987) *Developing Services for People with Severe Learning Difficulties and Challenging Behaviours*, Canterbury: Institute of Social and Applied Psychology

Emerson, E. and Hatton, C. (2004) *Estimating the Current Need/Demand for Supports for People with Learning Disabilities in England*, Lancaster: Institute for Health Research, Lancaster University.

Emerson, E. and Hatton, C. (2007a) *The Mental Health of Children and Adolescents with Learning Disabilities in Britain*, Lancaster: Institute for Health Research, Lancaster University.

Emerson E. and Hatton, C. (2007b) 'Contribution of socioeconomic position to health inequalities of British children and adolescents with intellectual disabilities', *American Journal on Mental Retardation*, 112: 140–50.

Emerson, E. and Hatton, C. (2009) *Estimating Future Need for Adult Social Care Services for People with Learning Disabilities in England*, Centre for Disability Research Report, http://eprints.lancs.ac.uk/21049/1/CeDR

Emerson, E., R. Madden, *et al.* (2009) *Intellectual and Physical Disability, Social Mobility, Social Inclusion and Health*, Lancaster University, Centre for Disability Research.

Emerson, E., Malam, S. *et al.* (2005) *Adults with Learning Difficulties in England 2003/4: Full Report*, Leeds: NHS Health and Social Care Information Centre.

Emerson, E. and Robertson, J. (2008) *Commissioning Person-Centred, Cost-Effective, Local Support for People with Learning Disabilities*, SCIE Knowledge Review 20, London: SCIE.

Emerson, E., Robertson, J. Gregory, N. *et al.* (2001) 'Quality and costs of supported living residences and group homes in the UK', *American Journal on Mental Retardation*, 106: 401–15.

Ericsson, K. (2002) *From Institutional Life to Community Participation: Ideas and Realities Concerning Support to Persons with Intellectual Disability*, Uppsala: Uppsala University.

Everitt, G. and Williams, V. (2007) *Have Your Say about College: A Report on FE Provision for Young People with Learning Disabilities in Somerset*, Bristol: Norah Fry Research Centre.

Every Disabled Child Matters (2006) Campaign run by MENCAP, Contact a Family, Special Education Consortium and the Council for Disabled Children, www.edcm.org.uk

Farrell, P., Alborz, A., Howes, A. and Pearson, D. (2010) 'The impact of teaching assistants on improving pupils' academic achievement in mainstream schools: a review of the literature'. *Educational Review*, 62(4): 435–48.

Felce, D. and Emerson, E. (2001) 'Living with support in a home in the community: Predictors of behavioral development and household and community activity', *Mental Retardation and Developmental Disabilities Research Reviews*, 7: 75–83.

Felt, P. with Walker, P. (2000) 'My life in L'Arche', in R. Traustadottir and K. Johnson (eds), *Women with Intellectual Disabilities: Finding a Place in the World*, London: Jessica Kingsley, 217–28.

Finkelstein, V. (2004) 'Representing disability', in J. Swain, S. French, C. Barnes and C. Thomas (eds), *Disabling Barriers: Enabling Environments*, 2nd edn, London: Sage, 13–20.

Finlay, W. M. L., Antaki, C. and Walton, C. (2008) 'Saying no to the staff: an analysis of refusals in a home for people with severe communication difficulties', *Sociology of Health and Illness*, 30: 55–75.

Firth, H. and Rapley, M. (1990) *From Acquaintance to Friendship: Issues for People with Learning Disabilities*, Kidderminster: BIMH.

Fish R. and Culshaw, E. (2005) 'The last resort? Staff and client perspectives on physical intervention', *Journal of Intellectual Disabilities*, 9: 93–107.

Forbat, L. (2006) 'An analysis of key principles in valuing people: implications for supporting people with dementia', *Journal of Intellectual Disabilities*, 10: 249–60.

Forrester-Jones, R., Carpenter, J. *et al.* (2006) 'The social networks of people with intellectual disability living in the community 12 years after resettlement from long-stay hospitals', *Journal of Applied Research in Intellectual Disabilities*, 9(4): 285–95.

Forster, S. and Iacono, T. (2008) 'Disability support workers' experience of interaction with a person with profound intellectual disability', *Journal of Intellectual and Developmental Disability*, 33(2): 137–47.

Foster-Galasso, M. L. (2005) 'Diagnosis as an aid and a curse in dealing with others', in J. F. Duchan and D. Kovarsky (eds), *Diagnosis as Cultural Practice*, Berlin: Mouton de Gruyter, 17–32

Foucault, M. (1980) *Power/Knowledge: Selected Interviews and Other Writings 1972–1977*, London: Harvester Press.

Foundation for People with Learning Disabilities (2002) *Count Us In*, London: FPLD.

Fox, N. (ongoing) 'Inclusion in further education for students with communication difficulties', University of Bristol: Norah Fry Research Centre.

Frawley, P. (2008) *Participation in Government Disability Advisory Bodies: An Intellectual Disability Perspective*, Melbourne, Australia: LaTrobe University report for department of human services – disability services.

Frederickson, N. and Cline, T. (2002) *Special Educational Needs, Inclusion and Diversity*, Maidenhead: Open University Press.

Frost, N. (2005) *Professionalism, Partnership and Joined-up Thinking: A Research Review of Front-Line Working with Children and Families*, Devon: Research in Practice.

Fyson, R. (2009) 'Independence and learning disabilities: why we must also recognise vulnerability', *Journal of Integrated Care*, 17(1): 3–8.

Fyson, L. and Fox, L. (2008) *The Role and Effectiveness of Learning Disability Partnership Boards*, Nottingham: International Centre for Public and Social Policy.

Fyson, R., McBride, G. and Ward, L. (2004) 'How was it for you? Viewpoint', *Mencap*, 81: 14–17.

Fyson, R., Tarleton, B. and Ward, L. (2007) *The Impact of the Supporting People Programme on Housing and Support for Adults with Learning Disabilities*, Bristol: Policy Press, for Joseph Rowntree Foundation.

Gant, V. (2010) 'Older carers and adults with learning disabilities; stress and reciprocal care', *Mental Health and Learning Disabilities Research and Practice*, 7(2): 160–72.

Garvey, F. (2008) 'Setting up a learning disability liaison team in acute care', *Nursing Times*, 104(28): 30–1.

Geekie, P. and Raban, B. (1994) 'Language learning at home and school', in C. Gallaway and B. Richards, Input and Interaction in Language Acquisition, Cambridge: Cambridge University Press, 153–60

Giangreco, M. (2010) 'Utilization of teacher assistants in inclusive schools: is it the kind of help that helping is all about?', *European Journal of Special Needs Education*, 25(4): 341–5.

Gillman, M., Heyman, B. and Swain, J. (2000) 'What's in a name? The implications of diagnosis for people with learning difficulties and their family carers', *Disability and Society*, 15(3): 389–409.

Glasby, J. and Littlechild, R. (2009) *Direct Payments and Personal Budgets: Putting Personalisation into Practice*, Bristol: Policy Press.

Glazzard, J. (2011) 'Perceptions of the barriers to effective inclusion in one primary school: voices of teachers and teaching assistants', *Support for Learning*,26(2): 56–63.

Glendinning, C. *et al.* (2008), Evaluation of the Individual Budget Initiative (IBSEN), York: Social Policy Research Unit, University of York, http://php.york.ac.uk/inst/spru/research/summs/ibsen.php

Goffman, E. (1963) *Stigma: Notes on the Management of Spoiled Identity*, New Jersey, NJ: Prentice-Hall.

Goldbart, J. and Caton, S. (2009) *Communication and People with the Most Complex Needs: What Works and Why This Is Essential*, Report for Mencap, London: Mencap.

Goodley, D. (1997) Locating self-advocacy in models of disability: understanding disability in the support of self-advocates with learning difficulties. Disability and Society 12(3): 367–79.

Goodley, D. (2000) *Self-Advocacy in the Lives of People with Learning Difficulties*, Buckingham: Open University Press.

Goodley, D. (2011) *Disability Studies: An Interdisciplinary Introduction*, London: Sage

Goodley, D. and Norouzi, G. (2005) 'Enabling futures for people with learning difficulties? Exploring employment realities behind the policy rhetoric', in A. Roulstone and C. Barnes (eds), *Working Future? Disabled People, Policy and Social Inclusion*, Bristol: Policy Press, 219–31.

Gorfin, L., McGlaughlin, A. and Saul, C. (2004) 'Enabling adults with learning disabilities to articulate their housing needs', *British Journal of Social Work*, 34: 709–26.

Government Response to the Education and Skills Committee report on Special Educational Needs (2006), London: TSO.

Gramlich, S., McBride, G. and Snelham, N. with Williams, V. and Simons, K. (2002) *Journey to Independence: What Self-Advocates Tell Us about Direct Payments*, Kidderminster: BILD.

Grant, G., Goward, P., Richardson, M. and Ramcharan, P. (eds) (2010) *Learning Disability: A Life Cycle Approach to Valuing People*, 2nd edn, Buckingham: Open University Press.

Greatbatch, D. and Dingwall, R. (1998) 'Talk and identity in divorce mediation', in C. Antaki and S. Widdicombe (eds) *Identities in Talk*, London: Sage.

Grey, I., Hastings, R. and McClean, B. (2007) 'Staff training and challenging behaviour', *Journal of Applied Research in Intellectual Disabilities*, 20(1): 1–5.

Guinea, S. (2001) 'Parents with a learning disability and their views on support received: a preliminary study', *Journal of Learning Disabilities*, 5: 43–6.

Gurit, L. and Ells, C. (2010) 'Adults with intellectual and developmental disabilities and participation in decision making: ethical considerations for professional-client practice', *Intellectual and Developmental Disabilities*, 48(2): 112–25.

Hall, I., Strydom, A., Richards *et al.* (2005) 'Social outcomes in adulthood of children with intellectual impairment: evidence from a birth cohort', *Journal of Intellectual Disability Research*, 49: 171–82.

Hall, L. and Hewson, S. (2006) 'The community links of a sample of people with intellectual disabilities', *Journal of Applied Research in Intellectual Disabilities*, 19: 204–7.

Hannon, L. (2004) 'Better preadmission assessment improves learning disability care', *Nursing Times*, 100: 44–7.

Harman, A. and Sanderson, H. (2008) 'How person-centred is active support?', *Journal of Intellectual and Developmental Disability*, 33(3): 271–3.

Harris, J. R. (2000) 'Socialization, personality development, and the child's environments: comment on Vandell', *Developmental Psychology*, 36(6), 699–710.

Hartas, D. and Lindsay, G. (2011) 'Young people's involvement in service evaluation and decision making', *Emotional and Behavioural Difficulties*,16(2): 129–43.

Hassiotis, A., Robotham, D., Canagasabey, A. *et al.* (2009) 'Randomized, single-blind, controlled trial of a specialist behaviour therapy team for challenging behavior in adults with intellectual disabilities', *American Journal of Psychiatry*, 166: 1278–85.

Hatton, C. (2002) 'Psychosocial interventions for adults with intellectual disabilities and mental health problems: a review', *Journal of Mental Health*, 11: 357–73.

Hatton, C., Akram, Y., Shah, R. *et al.* (2004) *Supporting South Asian Families with a Child with Severe Disabilities*, London: Jessica Kingsley.

Hatton, C. and Emerson, E. (1996) *Residential Provision for People with Learning Disabilities: A Research Review*, Manchester: Hester Adrian Research Centre. www.lancs.ac.uk/shm/dhr/research/learning/publications/residential.htm

Hatton, C. R., Robertson, J., Shah, R. and Akram, Y. (2004a) *Supporting South Asian Families with a Child with Severe Disabilities*, London: Jessica Kingsley.

Hatton, C., Emerson, E., Robertson, J. *et al.* (2004b) 'The Resident Choice Scale: a measure to assess opportunities for self-determination in residential settings', *Journal of Intellectual Disability Research*, 48: 103–13.

Hawkins, S. Allen, D. and Jenkins, R. (2005) 'The use of physical interventions with people with intellectual disabilities and challenging behaviour: the experiences of service users and staff members', *Journal of Applied Research in Intellectual Disabilities*, 18: 19–34.

Hayashi, R. and Okuhira, M. (2008) 'The independent living movement in Asia: solidarity from Japan', *Disability and Society*, 23(5): 417–30.

Helen Sanderson Associates, CSIP, Valuing People, in Control, London Borough of Newham (2010) *After School, What's possible?* DVD available from www.hsapress.co.uk/publications/dvd's.aspx

Heller, T. and Arnold, C. (2010) 'Siblings of adults with developmental disabilities: psychosocial outcomes, relationships, and future planning', *Journal of Policy and Practice in Intellectual Disabilities*, 7(1): 16–25.

Heslop, P. (2006) *Medication Matters*, Bristol: Norah Fry Research Centre.

Heslop, P. *et al.* (2002) *Bridging the Divide at Transition: What Happens for Young People with Learning Difficulties and Their Families?*, Bristol: Norah Fry Research Centre.

Heslop, P., Abbott, D., Johnson, L. and Mallett, R. (2007) *Help to Move on: Transition Pathways for Young People with Learning Difficulties in Residential Schools and Colleges*, Bristol: Norah Fry Research Centre.

Heslop, P. and Macaulay, F. (2009) *Hidden Pain: Self-Injury and People with Learning Disabilities*, Bristol: Norah Fry Research Centre.

Hill, C. and Rose, J. (2009) 'Parenting stress in mothers of adults with an intellectual disability: parental cognitions in relation to child characteristics and family support', *Journal of Intellectual Disability Research*, 53(12): 969–80.

Hiscoe, C. with Johnson, K. (2007) 'Be there for me: case management in my life', in C. Bigby, C. Fyffe and E. Ozanne (eds), *Planning and Support for People with Intellectual Disabilities: Issues for Case Managers and Other Professionals*, London: Jessica Kingsley, 162–70.

Holloway, D. (2004) 'Ethical dilemmas in community learning disability nursing: what helps resolve ethical dilemmas that result from choices made by people with learning disabilities?' *Journal of Learning Disabilities*, 8: 283.

Hornby, G. and Ravleen, L. (2011) 'Barriers to parental involvement in education: an explanatory model', *Educational Review*, 63(1): 37.

Hortham Memories Group (1994) *Hortham Memories*, Bristol: South Bristol College (available from Norah Fry Research Centre, University of Bristol).

Houghton, M. (2010) *A Step by Step Guide for GP Practices: Annual Health Checks for People with a Learning Disability*, London: Royal College of General Practitioners.

House of Commons Education and Skills Committee (2006) *Special Educational Needs: Third Report of Session 2005–6: Vol. 1*, www.publications.parliament.uk/pa/ cm200506/cmselect/cmeduski/478/478i.pdf

Hubert J. (2006) 'Family carers' views of services for people with learning disabilities from Black and minority ethnic groups: a qualitative study of 30 families in a south London borough', *Disability and Society*, 21(3): 259–72.

Hunter S. and Ridley, J. (2007), 'Supported employment in Scotland: some issues from research and implications for development', *Tizard Learning Disability Review*, 12(2): 3–13.

Hunter, S. and Ritchie, P. (eds) (2007) *Co-Production and Personalisation in Social Care: Changing Relationships in the Provision of Social Care*, London: Jessica Kingsley.

Jacobsen, Y. (2002) *Making the Jump*, Leicester, National Institute for Adult and Continuing Education.

Jacobsen, Y. (2005) *Person-Centred Planning and Post-16 Education*, Leicester, National Institute for Adult and Continuing Education.

Jahoda, A. and Wanless, L. K. (2005) 'Knowing you: the interpersonal perceptions of staff towards aggressive individuals with mild to moderate intellectual disabilities in situations of conflict', *Journal of Intellectual Disability Research*, 49: 544–51.

James, H. (2004), 'Promoting effective working with parents with learning disabilities', *Child Abuse Review*, 13: 31–41.

Jenner, P. and Gale, T. M. (2006) 'A relationship support service for people with learning disabilities', *Learning Disability Review*, 11: 18–25.

Jepson, M. (2011) 'Who decides? Decision making with people with learning disabilities under the Mental Capacity Act 2005, Ph.D. thesis, University of Bristol.

Jingree, T., Finlay, W. M. L. and Antaki, C. (2006) 'Empowering words, disempowering actions: an analysis of interactions between staff members and people with learning disabilities in residents' meetings', *Journal of Intellectual Disability Research*, 50(3): 212–26.

Johnson, K. (1998) *Deinstitutionalising Women: An Ethnographic Study of Institutional Closure*, Melbourne: Cambridge University Press

Johnson, K. (2000a) 'Finding a place', in R. Traustadottir and K. Johnson (eds), *Women with Intellectual Disabilities: Finding a Place in the World*, London: Jessica Kingsley, 9–24.

Johnson, K. (2000b) 'In the world', in R. Traustadottir and K. Johnson (eds), *Women with Intellectual Disabilities: Finding a Place in the World*, London: Jessica Kingsley, 271–9.

Johnson, K. (2010) 'A late picking: narratives of older people with learning disabilities', in G. Grant, P. Goward, M. Richardson and P. Ramcharan (eds), *Learning Disability: A Life Cycle Approach to Valuing People*, Milton Keynes: Open University Press, 647–62.

Johnson, K., Hillier, L., Harrison, L. and Frawley, P. (2001) *People with Intellectual Disabilities: Safer Sexual Lives*, Melbourne: Latrobe University.

Johnson, K. and Traustadottir, R. (2005) *In and Out of Institutions: Deinstitutionalisation in the Twenty First Century*, London: Jessica Kingsley.

Johnson, K., Walmsley, J. and Wolfe, M. (2010) *People with Intellectual Disabilities: Towards a Good Life*, Bristol: Policy Press.

Joint Committee on Human Rights (2008) *A Life Like Any Other? Human Rights of Adults with Learning Disabilities*, House of Commons HL Paper 40–II, London: TSO.

Jones, P. and Stenfert-Kroese, B. (2007) 'Service users' views of physical restraint procedures in secure settings for people with learning disabilities', *British Journal of Learning Disabilities*, 35: 50–4.

Jones, E. and Lowe, K. (2008) 'Active support is person-centred by definition: a response to Harman and Sanderson', *Journal of Intellectual and Developmental Disability*, 33(3): 274–7.

Jones, P. (2010) 'My peers have also been an inspiration for me: developing online learning opportunities to support teacher engagement with inclusive pedagogy for students with severe/profound intellectual developmental disabilities', *International Journal of Inclusive Education*, 14(7): 681–96.

Joyce, T. and Shuttleworth, L. (2001) 'From engagement to participation: how do we bridge the gap?', *British Journal of Learning Disabilities*, 29: 63–71.

Kaehne, A. (2010) 'Multiagency protocols in intellectual disabilities transition partnerships: a survey of local authorities in Wales', *Journal of Policy and Practice in Intellectual Disabilities*, 7(3): 182–8.

Kalambouka, A., Farrell, P., Dyson, A. and Kaplan, I. (2007) 'The impact of placing pupils with special educational needs in mainstream schools on the achievement of their peers', *Educational Research*, 49(4): 365–82.

Kaplan, R. (2010) 'Caregiving mothers of children with impairments: coping and support in Russia', *Disability and Society*, 25(6): 715–30.

Kellett, M. (2011) *Children's Perspectives on Integrated Services*, Basingstoke: Palgrave Macmillan.

Kerr, M. and Bowley, C. (2001) 'Evidence-based prescribing in adults with learning disability and epilepsy', *Epilepsia*, 42 (Suppl. 1): 44–5.

Kerr, M., Cunningham, C. and Wilkinson, H. (2006) 'Learning disability and dementia: are we prepared?', *Journal of Dementia*, Care May/June: 17–19.

Kerr, M., Fraser, W. and Felce, D. (2009) 'Primary health care for people with a learning disability: a keynote review', *British Journal of Learning Disabilities*, 24(1): 2–8.

King, N. and Abbey, D. (2010) *Ownership Options for People with a Learning Disability*, London: NHF.

Knott, F. Dunlop, A. W. and Mackay, T. (2006) 'Living with ASD: how do children and their parents assess their difficulties with social interaction and understanding?', *Autism*, 10: 609–17.

Lacey, P. (2001) *Support Partnerships: Collaboration in Action*, London: David Fulton.

Langan, M. (2011) 'Parental voices and controversies in autism', *Disability and Society*, 26(2): 193–205.

Learning and Skills Council (2005) *Through Inclusion to Excellence*, London: LSC.

Learning and Skills Council (2006) *Learning for Living and Work: Improving Education and Training Opportunities for people with Learning Difficulties and/or Disabilities*, London: LSC.

Lennox, T., Nadkarni, J., Moffat, O. and Robertson, C. (2003) 'Access to services and meeting the needs of people with learning disabilities', *Journal of Learning Disabilities*, 7: 34–50.

Lindsay, G. (2003) 'Inclusive education: a critical perspective', *British Journal of Special Education*, 30(1): 3–12.

Lindsay, G. (2007) 'Educational psychology and the effectiveness of inclusion/mainstreaming', *British Journal of Educational Psychology*, 77: 1–29.

Lunt, J. and Hinz, A. (eds) (2011) *Training and Practice in Person Centred Planning: A European Perspective*, Stamford: New Paths.

McCarthy, M. (1999) *Sexuality and Women with Learning Disabilities*, London: Jessica Kingsley Publishers.

McCarthy, M. (2010) 'What kind of future for young people with Down's syndrome? The views and aspirations of young people and families', *Tizard Learning Disability Review*, 15(4): 30–3.

McConkey, R. McConaghie, J. Mezza, F. and Wilson, J. (2003) 'Moving from long-stay hospitals: the views of Northern Irish patients and relatives', *Journal of Learning Disabilities*, 7: 78–93.

McConkey, R. (1998) 'Community integration and ordinary lifestyles', in P. Lacey and C. Ouvry (eds), *People with Profound and Multiple Learning Disabilities: A Collaborative Approach to Meeting Complex Needs*, London: David Fulton, 184–93.

McConkey, R. and Collins, S. (2010) 'The role of support staff in promoting the social inclusion of persons with an intellectual disability', *Journal of Intellectual Disability Research*, 54(8): 691–700.

McConnell, D., Llewellyn, G., Traustadottir, R. and Sigurjonsdottir, H. B. (2010) 'Conclusion: taking stock and looking to the future', in G. Llewellyn, R. Traustadottir, D. McConnell and H. B. Sigurjonsdottir (eds), *Parents with Intellectual Disabilities: Past, Present and Futures*, Chichester: Wiley, 240–57.

McCormack, B. and Farrell, M. (2009) 'Translating quality of life into service action: use of personal outcome measures in the Republic of Ireland', *British Journal of Learning Disabilities*, 37: 300–7.

MacDonald, E. and Hastings, P. (2010) 'Mindful parenting and care involvement of fathers of children with intellectual disabilities', *Journal of Child and Family Studies*, 19(2): 236.

McGaw, S. and Newman, T. (2005) *What works for Parents with Learning Disabilities*, Ilford: Barnardo's.

McKenzie, K. (2011) 'Providing services in the United Kingdom to people with an intellectual disability who present behaviour which challenges. A review of the literature', *Research in Developmental Disabilities*, 32: 395–403.

McKenzie, K., Broad, R., McLean, H., Wilson, S., Megson, P. and Miller, S. (2009) 'Evaluating a community-based project for supporting clients with challenging behaviour', *Learning Disability Practice*, 12(4): 27–32.

McKenzie, K., Powell, H. and McGregor, L. (2004) 'The impact of control and restraint training on nursing students', *Learning Disability Practice*, 7: 34–7.

McLaughlin, D. F., Taggart, L. Quinn, B. and Milligan, V. (2007) 'The experiences of professionals who care for people with intellectual disability who have substance-related problems', *Journal of Substance Misuse*, 12: 133–43.

Mak, W. W. S. and Ho, G. S. M. (2007) 'Caregiving perceptions of Chinese mothers of children with intellectual disability in Hong Kong', *Journal of Applied Research in Intellectual Disabilities*, 20(2): 145–56.

Mansell, J. (2007) *Services for People with Learning Disabilities and Challenging Behaviour or Mental Health Needs: Out of Area Placements*, London: Department of Health.

Mansell, J. (2010) *Raising our Sights: Services for Adults with Profound Intellectual and Multiple Disabilities*, www.dh.gov.uk/en/Publicationsandstatistics

Mansell, J., Ashman, B. Macdonald, S. and Beadle-Brown, J. (2002a) 'Residential care in the community for adults with intellectual disability: needs characteristics and services', *Journal of Intellectual Disability Research*, 46: 625–33.

Mansell, J. and Beadle-Brown, J. (2004) 'Person-centred planning or person-centred action? Policy and practice in intellectual disability services', *Journal of Applied Research in Intellectual Disabilities*, 17: 1–9.

Mansell, J., Beadle-Brown, J., Cambridge, P. *et al.* (2009) 'Adult protection', *Journal of Social Work*, 9(1): 23.

Mansell, J., Elliott, T., Beadle-Brown, J., Ashman, B. and Macdonald, S. (2002b) 'Engagement in meaningful activity and "active support" of people with intellectual disabilities in residential care', *Research in Developmental Disabilities*, 23(5), 342–52.

Marriott, A. and Williams, V. (2011) 'Inclusive research: people with learning disabilities can be the "artists of their lives"', in H. Atherton and D. Crickmore (eds), *Learning Disability: Towards Inclusion*, London: Elsevier, 161–77.

Mansell, I. and Wilson, C. (2010) '"It terrifies me, the thought of the future": listening to the current concerns of informal carers of people with a learning disability', *Journal of Intellectual Disabilities*, 14(1): 21–31.

Marshall, D., McConkey, R. and Moore, G. (2003) 'Obesity in people with intellectual disabilities: the impact of nurse-led health screenings and health promotion activities', *Journal of Advanced Nursing*, 41: 147–53.

Marshall, T. H. (1950) *Citizenship and Social Class*, Cambridge: Cambridge University Press.

Martin, G. (2003) 'Annual health reviews for patients with severe learning disabilities', *Journal of Learning Disabilities*, 7: 9–21.

Maye, R. and Sigurjonsdottir, H. B. (2010) 'Becoming a mother – becoming a father', in G. Llewellyn, R. Traustadottir, D. McConnell and H. B. Sigurjonsdottir (eds), *Parents with Intellectual Disabilities: Past, Present and Futures*, Chichester: Wiley, 17–32.

Melville, C. A., Hamilton, S., Hankey, C. R., Miller, S. and Boyle, S. (2007) 'The prevalence and determinants of obesity in adults with intellectual disabilities', *Obesity Reviews*, 8: 223–30.

Mencap (2004) *PMLD Network – Partnership Board Survey 2004*, London: Mencap.

Mencap (2007) *Death by Indifference*, www.mencap.org.uk/node/5863 (accessed April 2012).

Mencap (2008) *Profound and Multiple Learning Disability definition*, www.mencap.org.uk/document.asp?id=539 (accessed 8 August 2010).

Mencap (2012) *Death by Indifference: 74 Deaths and Counting*, www.mencap.org.uk/74deaths (accessed April 2012).

Mepham, S. (2010) 'Disabled children: the right to feel safe', *Child Care in Practice*, 16(1): 19–34.

Miles, S. and Singal, N. (2010) 'The education for all and inclusive debate: conflict, contradiction or opportunity?', *Journal of Inclusive Education* ,14(1): 1–15.

Millar, S. and Aitken, S. (2003) *Personal Communication Passports: Guidelines for Good Practice*, Edinburgh: Call Centre.

Millear, A. with Johnson, K. (2000) 'Thirty nine months under the Disability Discrimination Act', in R. Traustadottir and K. Johnson (eds), *Women with Intellectual Disabilities: Finding a Place in the World*, London: Jessica Kingsley, 239–52.

Milner, P. and Kelly. B. (2009) 'Community participation and inclusion: people with disabilities defining their place', *Disability and Society*, 24(1): 47–62.

Mitchell, W. (1999) 'Leaving special school: the next step and future aspirations', *Disability and Society*, 14: 753–69.

Mittler, P. (2008) 'Planning for the 2040s: everybody's business', British *Journal of Special Education*, 35(1): 3–10.

Morris, J. (2004) 'Independent living and community care: a disempowering framework', *Disability and Society*, 19(5): 427–42.

Morris, J. (2005) Citizenship and disabled people: a scoping paper prepared for the Disability Rights Commission. London: DRC.

Murphy, K., Cooney, K., Shea, E. and Casey, D. (2009) 'Determinants of quality of life for older people living with a disability in the community', *Journal of Advanced Nursing*, 65(3), 606–15.

Murray, P. (2000) 'Disabled children, parents and professionals: partnership on whose terms?', *Disability and Society*, 15(4): 683–98.

Murray, P. (2004) 'Participation: for a change: disabled young people lead the way', *Children and Society*, 18(2): 143–54.

Nellis, T. (1994) 'Self-advocacy: realizing a dream', *Impact*, 7(1): 1.

Nilholm, C. and Alm, B. (2010) 'An inclusive classroom? A case study of inclusiveness, teachers' strategies and children's experiences', *European Journal of Special Needs Education*, 25(3): 239–52.

Nind, M., Flewitt, R. and Payler, J. (2010) 'The social experience of early childhood for children with learning disabilities: inclusion, competence and agency', *British Journal of Sociology of Education*, 31(6): 653–70.

Nirje, B. (1969) 'The normalization principle and its human management implications', in R. Kugel and W. Wolfensberger (eds), *Changing Patterns in Residential Services for the Mentally Retarded*, Washington DC: Presidential Committee on Mental Retardation.

Noonan-Walsh, P., Linehan, C., Hillery, J. *et al.* (2001) 'Family views of the quality of residential supports', *Journal of Applied Research in Intellectual Disabilities*, 14: 292–309.

Norwich, B. (2002) 'Education, inclusion and individual differences: Recognising and resolving dilemmas', *British Journal of Educational Studies*, 50(4): 482–502.

O'Brien, C. L. and O'Brien, J. (2000) 'The origins of person-centred planning: a community of practice perspective', in S. Holburn and P. Vietze (eds), *Person-Centred Planning: Research, Practice, and Future Directions*, Baltimore, MD: Paul H. Brookes.

O'Brien, J., Pearpoint, J. and Kahn, L. (2010) *The PATH and MAPS Handbook: Person-Centered Ways to Build Community*, Toronto: Inclusion Press.

Office for Disability Issues (2008) *The Independent Living Strategy*, London: TSO.

Ofsted (2004) *Special Educational Needs and Disability: Towards Inclusive Schools*, London: Ofsted.

Ofsted (2010) *The Special Educational Needs and Disability Review: A Statement Is Not Enough*, London: Ofsted.

O'Hara, J. and Martin, H. (2003) 'Parents with learning disabilities: a study of gender and cultural perspectives in East London', *British Journal of Learning Disabilities*, 31: 18–24.

Oliver, M. (1990) *The Politics of Disablement*, Butterworth: Heinemann.

Oliver, M. (1992) 'Changing the social relations of research production?', *Disability, Handicap and Society*, 7(2): 101–14.

Oliver, M. (2004) 'If I had a hammer', in J. Swain, S. French, C. Barnes and C. Thomas (eds), *Disabling Barriers – Enabling Environments*, 2nd edn, London: Sage, 1–12.

Osborne, L. and Reed, P. (2011) 'School factors associated with mainstream progress in secondary education for included pupils with autism spectrum disorders', *Research in Autism Spectrum Disorders*, 5(3): 1253–63.

Perry, J. (2004) 'Hate crime against people with learning difficulties: the role of the Crime and Disorder Act and no secrets in identification and prevention', *Journal of Adult Protection*, 6: 27–34.

Pilnick, A., Clegg, J., Murphy, E. and Almack, K. (2010) 'Questioning the answer: questioning style, choice and self-determination in interactions with young people with intellectual disabilities', *Sociology of Health and Illness*, 32(3): 415–36.

Pilnick, A., Clegg, J., Murphy, E. and Almack, K. (2011) '"Just being selfish for my own sake…": balancing the views of young adults with intellectual disabilities and their carers in transition planning', *Sociological Review*, 59(2): 303–23.

PIRU (Public Interest Research Unit) (2005) *The End of the Beginning: An Analysis of the First Decade of the Disability Discrimination Act Employment Provisions (1995–2005)*, www.piru.org.uk/press-releases/ten-years-of-dda

Pockney, R. (2006) 'Friendship or facilitation: people with learning disabilities and their paid carers', *Sociological Research Online*, www.socresonline.org.uk/11/3/pockney.html

Poll, C. (2007) 'Co-production in supported housing: KeyRing Living Support Networks and neighbourhood networks', in S. Hunter and P. Ritchie (eds), *Co-Production and Personalisation in Social Care: Changing Relationships in the Provision of Social Care*, London: Jessica Kingsley, 49–66.

Ponting, L., Ford, K. and the Skills for Support Team (2010) *Training Personal Assistants*, Brighton: Pavilion Publishing.

Porter, J., Ouvry, C., Morgan, M. and Downs, C. (2001) 'Interpreting the communication of people with profound and multiple learning difficulties', *British Journal of Learning Disabilities*, 29: 12–16.

Potter, J. (2003) 'Discursive psychology: between method and paradigm', *Discourse and Society*, 14: 783–94.

Prime Minister's Strategy Unit (2005) *Improving the Life Chances of Disabled People*, London: TSO.

Prime Minister's Strategy Unit (2007) Building on Progress: Public Services, HM Government Policy Review, London: TSO.

Raghavan, R., Waseem, N., Small, N. and Newell, R. (2005) 'Supporting young people with learning disabilities and mental health needs from minority ethnic groups', in *Making us Count: Identifying and Improving Mental Health Support for Young People with Learning Disabilities*, London: Foundation for People with Learning Disabilities.

Ramcharan, P., Roberts, G., Grant, G. and Borland, J. (1997) *Empowerment in Everyday Life: Learning Disability*, London: Jessica Kingsley.

Randell, M. and Cumella, S. (2009) 'People with an intellectual disability living in an intentional community', *Journal of Intellectual Disability Research*, 53(8): 716–26.

Rao, S. (2006) 'Parameters of normality and cultural constructions of "mental retardation": perspectives of Bengali families', *Disability and Society*, 21(2): 159–78.

Rapley, M. (2004) *The Social Construction of Learning Disability*, Cambridge: Cambridge University Press.

Rapley, M., Kiernan, P. and Antaki, C. (1998) 'Invisible to themselves or negotiating identity? The interactional management of "being intellectually disabled"', *Disability and Society*, 13(5): 807–27.

Redley, M. and Weinberg, D. (2007) 'Learning disability and the limits of liberal citizenship: interactional impediments to political empowerment', *Sociology of Health and Illness*, 29(5): 1–20.

Redley, M. (2009) 'Understanding the social exclusion and stalled welfare of citizens with learning disabilities', *Disability and Society*, 24(4), 498–501.

Reynolds F. (2002) 'An exploratory survey of opportunities and barriers to creative leisure activity for people with learning disabilities', *British Journal of Learning Disabilities*, 30: 63–7.

Richardson, M. (2010) 'Critiques of segregation and eugenics', in G. Grant, P. Goward, M. Richardson and P. Ramcharan (eds), *Learning Disability: A Life Cycle Approach to Valuing People*, Maidenhead: Open University Press, ch. 4.

Riddington, C., Mansell, J. and Beadle–Brown, J. (2008) 'Are partnership boards really valuing people?', *Disability and Society*, 23(6): 649–66.

Riggins, S. (ed.) (1997) *The Language and Politics of Exclusion: Others in Discourse*, London: Sage.

Rioux, M. and Bach, M. (1994) *Disability is Not Measles: New Research Paradigms In Disability*, North York: Roeher Institute.

Ritchie, P., Sanderson, H., Kilbane, J. and Routledge, M. (2003) *People, Plans and Practicalities: Achieving Change through Person Centred Planning*, Manchester: Helen Sanderson Associates.

Rix, J. and Paige-Smith, A. (2008) 'A different head? Parental agency and early intervention', *Disability and Society*, 23(3): 211–22.

Robertson, J., Emerson, E., Gregory, N. *et al.* (2001a) 'Social networks of people with mental retardation in residential settings', *Mental Retardation*, 39: 201–14.

Robertson, J., Emerson, E., Gregory, N. *et al.* (2001b) 'Environmental opportunities and supports for exercising self-determination in community-based residential settings', *Research in Developmental Disabilities*, 22: 487–502.

Robertson, J., Emerson, E., Hatton, C. *et al.* (2005) *The Impact of Person Centred Planning*, Lancaster: Institute for Health Research, Lancaster University.

Robertson, J., Emerson, E., Hatton, C. *et al.* (2007a) 'Person-centred planning: factors associated with successful outcomes for people with intellectual disabilities', *Journal of Intellectual Disability Research*, 51(3): 232–43.

Robertson, J., Emerson, E., Hatton, C. *et al.* (2007b) 'Reported barriers to the implementation of person-centred planning for people with intellectual disabilities in the UK', *Journal of Applied Research in Intellectual Disabilities*, 20: 297–307.

Robertson, J., Roberts, H. and Emerson, E. (2010) *Health Checks for People with Learning Disabilities: A Systematic Review of Evidence*, Lancaster: Learning Disabilities Observatory.

Rodgers, J., Townsley, R., Tarleton, B., Folkes, L. and Mears, C. (2004) *Information for All: Guidance*, http://easyinfo.org.uk/index.jsp

Rogers, C. (2004) *On Becoming a Person: A Therapist's View of Psychotherapy*, London: Constable and Robinson.

Rogers, C. (2010) 'But it's not all about sex: mothering, normalisation and young learning disabled people', *Disability and Society*, 25(1): 63–74.

Rolph, S., Atkinson, D., Nind, M. and Welshman, J. (eds) (2005). *Witnesses to Change: Families, Learning Difficulties and History*, Buckingham: Open University Press.

Roulstone, A. and Prideaux, S. (2012) *Understanding Disability Policy*, Bristol: Policy Press.

Ruddick, L. and Oliver, C. (2005) 'The development of a health status measure for self-report by people with intellectual disabilities', *Journal of Applied Research in Intellectual Disabilities*, 18: 143–50.

Runswick-Cole, K. (2007) '"The Tribunal was the most stressful thing: more stressful than my son's diagnosis or behaviour": the experiences of families who go to the Special Educational Needs and Disability Tribunal (SENDisT)', *Disability and Society*, 22(3): 315–28.

Russell, F. (2011) Audit of the extent of Portage provision in England. NPA and DfE: www.portage.org.uk

Samuel, M. (2010) 'What price work? The future of employment support for people with disabilities', *Community Care* (26/08/10).

Sanderson, H. (2000) *Person Centred Planning: Key Features and Approaches*, York: Joseph Rowntree Foundation.

Sanderson, H., Kennedy, J., Ritchie, P. with Goodwin, G. (1999) *People Plans and Possibilities: Exploring Person Centred Planning*, Stockpot: Inclusion Distribution.

Sanderson, H. and Neil, M. (2009) *From Individual to Strategic Change: Driving Change with Person Centered Information*, Manchester: Helen Sanderson Associates.

Sarbin, T. and Kitsuse, J. (1994) 'A prologue to constructing the social', in T. Sarbin and J. Kitsuse (eds), *Constructing the Social*, London: Sage, 1–16.

Schelly, D. (2008) 'Problems associated with quality of life for an individual with intellectual disability: a personal assistant's reflexive ethnography', *Disability and Society*, 23(7): 719–32.

SCIE (2005) *Implementing the Carers (Equal Opportunities) Act 2004* (SCIE Guide 9)

Seligman, M. E. P. (1975) *Helplessness: On Depression, Development, and Death*, San Francisco, CA: W. H. Freeman.

Shah, A. (2010) 'The concept of "best interests" in the treatment of mentally incapacitated adults', *Journal of Forensic Psychiatry and Psychology*, 21(2): 306–16.

Shakespeare, T. (2006) *Disability Rights and Wrongs*, London: Routledge.

Shakespeare, T. and Watson, N. (1998) 'Theoretical perspectives on research with disabled children', in C. Robinson and K. Stalker (eds), *Growing up with Disability* (eds), London: Jessica Kingsley, 13–28.

Shearn, J. and Todd, S. (1997) 'Parental work: an account of the day to day activities of parents of adults with learning disabilities', *Journal of Intellectual Disability Research*, 41(4): 285–301.

Sigurjonsdottir, H. B. (2000) 'Motherhood, family and community life', in R. Traustadottir and K. Johnson (eds), *Women with Intellectual Disabilities: Finding a Place in the World*, London: Jessica Kingsley, 253–70.

Simons, K. (1998) *Living Support Networks: An Evaluation of the Services Provided by KeyRing*, Brighton: Pavilion Publishing.

Simons, K. (1999) *A Place at the Table? Involving People with Learning Difficulties in Purchasing and Commissioning Services*, Kidderminster: BILD.

Simons, K. (2000) *Pushing Open the Door. Housing Options: The Impact of a 'Housing and Support' Advisory Service*, Oxford: Marston Book Services.

Simons, K. and Ward, L. (1997) *A Foot in the Door: A Review of Supported Living for People with Learning Difficulties*, Manchester: National Development Team.

Simons, K. and Watson, D. (2002) *New Directions? Day Services for People with Learning Disabilities in the 1990s. A Review of the Research*, Exeter: Centre for Evidence based Social Services, University of Exeter.

Singal, N. (2010) 'Doing disability research in a Southern context: challenges and possibilities', *Disability and Society*, 25(4): 415–26.

Skills for Support Team (2005) *Getting Good Support*. Report of a survey. Available at Norah Fry Research Centre website.

Skinner, D. and Weisner, T. (2007) 'Sociocultural studies of families of children with intellectual disabilities', *Mental Retardation and Developmental Disabilities Research Reviews*, 13: 302–12.

Slattery, J. with Johnson, K. (2000) 'Family, marriage, friends and work: this is my life', in R. Traustadottir and K. Johnson (eds), *Women With Intellectual Disabilities: Finding a Place in the World*, London: Jessica Kingsley, 90–105.

Slee, R. (2010) 'Revisiting the politics of special educational needs and disability studies in education with Len Barton', *British Journal of Sociology of Education*, 31(5): 561–73.

Smith, N., Middleton, S., Ashton-Brooks, K., Cos, L., Dobson, B. with Reith, L. (2004) *Disabled People's Costs of Living: More than You Would Think*, York: Joseph Rowntree Foundation (available at: www.jrf.org.uk/bookshop/details.asp?pubID=635).

Social Care Institute for Excellence (2004) *SCIE Position Paper 3: Has Service User Participation Made a Difference to Social Care Services?* London: SCIE.

Society for Disability Studies (accessed 2012) Guidelines for Disability Studies Programmes. http://disstudies.org/guidelines-for-disability-studies-programs

Souza, A. with Ramcharam, P. (1997) 'Everything you ever wanted to know about Down's syndrome, but never bothered to ask', in P. Ramcharan, G. Roberts, G. Grant and J. Borland (eds), *Empowerment in Everyday Life: Learning Disability*, Jessica Kingsley: London.

Springate, I., Atkinson, M. *et al.* (2008) *Narrowing the Gap in Outcomes: Early Years (0–5 years)*, London: National Foundation for Educational Research.

Stalker, K and Connors, C. (2007) 'Children's experiences of disability: pointers to a social model of childhood disability', *Disability and Society*, 22(1): 19–34.

Stancliffe, R., Jones, E. and Mansell, J. (2008) 'Research in active support', *Journal of Intellectual and Developmental Disability* 33(3): 194–5.

Starling, S., Willis, A., Dracup, M. Burton, M. and Pratt, C. (2006) 'Right to sight: accessing eye care for adults who are learning disabled', *Journal of Intellectual Disabilities*, 10: 337–55.

Strategic Planning and Development Unit (2001) *Sexuality Policy*, Hobart Tasmania.

Strydom, A., Livingstone, G., King, M. and Hassiotis, A. (2007) 'Prevalence of dementia in intellectual disability using different diagnostic criteria', *British Journal of Psychiatry*, 191: 150–7.

Strydom, A., Romeo, R., Perez-Achiaqa, N. *et al.* (2010) 'Service use and cost of mental disorder in older adults with intellectual disability', *British Journal of Psychiatry*, 196(2): 133–8.

Sutcliffe, J. (1992) *Integration for Adults with Learning Difficulties: Contexts and Debates*, Leicester: NIACE.

Sutcliffe, J. and Simons, K. (1994) *Self-Advocacy and Adults with Learning Difficulties*, Leicester: NIACE.

Swift, P. and Mattingly, M. (2009) *A Life in the Community: An Action Research Project Promoting Citizenship for People with High Support Needs*, London: Foundation for People with Learning Disabilities.

Taggart, L. McLaughlin, D. Quinn, B. and Milligan, V. (2006) 'An exploration of substance misuse in people with intellectual disabilities', *Journal of Intellectual Disability Research*, 50: 588–97.

Tajfel, H., Billig, M. G., Bundy, R. P. and Flament, C. (1971) 'Social categorization and intergroup behaviour', *European Journal of Social Psychology*, 1: 149–77.

Tarleton, B. (2004) 'The road ahead: Information for young people with learning difficulties, their families and supporters at transition', www.scie.org.uk/publications/tra/files/report.pdf

Tarleton, B. (2012) *An Introduction to Parents with Learning Difficulties*. Web resource on: http://www.bristol.ac.uk/wtwpn (accessed 3 April 2012).

Tarleton, B., Ward, L. and Howarth, J. (2006) *Finding the Right Support? A Review of Issues and Positive Practice in Supporting Parents with Learning Difficulties and Their Children*, London: Baring Foundation.

Taylor, K. and Dodd, K. (2003) 'Knowledge and attitudes of staff towards adult protection', *Journal of Adult Protection*, 5: 26–32.

Teachers' TV (2011) *It's Cool to be Different*, www.teachers.tv

Thomas, C. (2004) 'How is disability understood? An examination of sociological approaches', *Disability and Society*, 19: 569–83.

Thompson, D. (2002) 'Misplaced and forgotten: people with learning disabilities in residential homes for older people', *Housing, Care and Support*, 5(1): 19 – 22.

Todd, S. and Shearn, J. (1997) 'Family dilemmas and secrets: parents' disclosure of information to their adult offspring with learning disabilities', *Disability and Society*, 12(3): 341–66.

Tomlinson, C. (2012) Love is simply not enough. Tizard *Learning Disability Review*, 17 (1): 26–31.

Tomlinson, J. (1996) *Inclusive Learning: The Report of the Committee of Enquiry into the Post-School Education of those with Learning Difficulties and/or Disabilities, in England*, London: HMSO.

Tomlinson, S. (2005) *Education in a Post-Welfare Society*, Buckingham: Open University Press.

Towers, C. (2009) *Recognising Fathers: A National Survey of Fathers Who Have Children with Learning Disabilities*, London: Foundation for People with a Learning Disability.

Townsley, R. and Robinson, C. (1999) 'What rights for disabled children? Home enteral tube feeding in the community', *Children and Society*, 13: 48–60.

Townsley, R., Abbott, D. and Watson, D. (2004) *Making a Difference? Exploring the Impact of Multi-Agency Working on Disabled Children with Complex Healthcare Needs, Their Families and the Professionals Who Support Them*, Bristol: Policy Press.

Townsley, R., Howarth, J., LeGrys, P. and Macadam, M. (2002) *Getting Involved in Choosing Staff: A Resource Pack for Supporters, Trainers, and Staff Working with People Who Have Developmental Disabilities.* Brighton: Pavilion Publishing.

Townsley, R., Ward, L., Abbott, D. and Williams, V. (2009) *The Implementation of Policies Supporting Independent Living for Disabled People in Europe: Synthesis Report*, Utrecht: Academy Network of European Disability Experts.

Townson, L., Macauley, S., Harkness, E. *et al.* (2007) 'Research project on advocacy and autism', *Disability* and *Society*, 22(5): 523–36.

Traustadottir, R. and Sigurjonsdottir, H. B. (2010) 'Parenting and resistance: strategies in dealing with services and professionals', in G. Llewellyn, R. Traustadottir, D. McConnell and H. B. Sigurjonsdottir (eds), *Parents with Intellectual Disabilities: Past, Present and Futures*, Chichester: Wiley, 107–18.

Tucker, S., Sutherland, R., Alldis, K. *et al.* (2012) *Work in Progress.* Cornwall: Cornwall People First, www.cornwallpeoplefirst.com

Tynan, H. and Allen, D. (2002) 'The impact of service user cognitive level on carer attributions for aggressive behaviour', *Journal of Applied Research in Intellectual Disabilities*, 15: 213–23.

Tyrer, F. Smith, L. K. and McGrother, C. W. (2007) 'Mortality in adults with moderate to profound intellectual disability: a population-based study', *Journal of Intellectual Disability Research*, 51: 520–7.

Tyrer, P., Oliver-Africano, P. C., Ahmed, Z. *et al.* (2008) 'Risperidone, haloperidol and placebo in the treatment of aggressive challenging behaviour in patients with intellectual disability: a randomized controlled trial', *Lancet*, 371: 57–63.

UN High Commissioner (2008) Convention on the Rights of Persons with Disabilities and its Optional Protocol, www.un.org/disabilities/documents/ppt/crpdbasics.ppt

UNESCO (1994) The Salamanca Statement and Framework for Action on Special Needs Education, Paris: UNESCO.

United Nations (2007) United Nations Convention on the Rights of Persons with Disabilities, Geneva: UN.

UPIAS (Union of the Physically Impaired against Segregation) (1976) Fundamental Principles of Disability, London: UPIAS.

Urwick, J. and Elliott, J. (2010) 'International orthodoxy versus national realities: inclusive schooling and the education of children with disabilities in Lesotho', *Comparative Education*, 46(2): 137–50.

Vlaskamp, C. and van der Putten, A. (2009) 'Focus on interaction: the use of an individualized support program for persons with profound intellectual and multiple disabilities', *Research in Developmental Disabilities*, 30: 873–83.

Vygotsky, L. S. (1987) 'Thinking and speech', in L. S. Vygotsky, *Collected Works*, ed. R. Rieber and A. Carton; trans. N. Minick, New York: Plenum, vol. 1, 39–285 (first published 1934, 1960).

Wagemans, A., van Schrojenstein, H. Lantman-de-Valk, I. Tuffrey-Wijne, G. Widdershoven and Curfs, L. (2010) 'End-of-life decisions: an important theme in the care for people with intellectual disabilities', *Journal of Intellectual Disability Research*, 54(6): 516–24.

Walmsley, J. (1993) 'Contradictions in caring: reciprocity and interdependence', *Disability, Handicap and Society*, 8(2): 129–41.

Walmsley, J. (1997) 'Including people with learning difficulties: theory and practice', in L. Barton and M. Oliver (eds), Disability Studies: Past, Present and Future, Leeds: Disability Press.

Walmsley, J. (1999) 'Community and people with learning difficulties', in J. Swain and S. French (eds), *Therapy and Learning Difficulties: Advocacy, Participation and Partnership*, Oxford: Butterworth-Heinemann, 156–70.

Walmsley, J. (2001) 'Normalisation, emancipatory research and inclusive research in Learning Disability', *Disability and Society*, 16(2): 187–205.

Walmsley, J. and Johnson, K. (2003) *Inclusive Research with People with Learning Disabilities: Past, Present and Futures*, London: Jessica Kingsley.

Walmsley, J. and Mannon, H. (2009) 'Parents as co-researchers: a participatory action research initiative involving parents of people with intellectual disabilities in Ireland', *British Journal of Learning Disabilities*, 37(4): 271–6.

Walmsley, J. and Rolph, S. (2001) 'The Development of community care for people with learning difficulties 1913–1946', *Critical Social Policy*, 21(1): 59–80.

Warnock, M. (1978) *Special Educational Needs: Report of the Committee of Enquiry into the Education of Handicapped Children and Young People*, London: HMSO, www.educationeng-land.org.uk/documents/warnock

Watchman, K. (2012) 'At a crossroads in care: the role of dementia in the marginalisation of people with Down's syndrome and dementia', Ph.D. thesis, University of Edinburgh.

Watson, D., Williams, V. and Wickham, C. (2006a) '"It's about having a life, isn't it?": employability, discrimination and disabled people', in M. Carpenter, B. Freda and S. Speeden (eds), *Beyond the Workfare State: Labour Markets, Equality and Human Rights*, Bristol: Policy Press, 27–42.

Watson, D., Tarleton, B. and Feiler, A. (2006b) *Participation in Education: Full Report on the Findings from Research on the Involvement of Children with Little or no Verbal Communication*, Bristol: Norah Fry Research Centre.

Weddell, K. (2008) 'Confusion about inclusion: patching up or systems change?', *British Journal of Special Education*, 35(3): 127–35.

Welshman, J. and Walmsley, J. (eds) (2006) *Community Care in Perspective: Care, Control and Citizenship*, Basingstoke: Palgrave Macmillan.

Wendelborg, C. and Tossebro, J. (2010) 'Marginalisation processes in inclusive education in Norway: a longitudinal study of classroom participation', *Disability and Society*, 25(6): 701–14.

Wetherell, M. (1998) 'Positioning and interpretative repertoires: conversation analysis and post-structuralism in dialogue', *Discourse and Society*, 9(3): 387–412.

Wharton, S., Hames, A. and Milner, H. (2005) 'The accessibility of general NHS services for children with disabilities', *Child: Care, Health and Development*, 31: 275–82.

White, C., Holland, E., Marsland, D. and Oakes, P. (2003) 'The identification of environments and cultures that promote the abuse of people with intellectual disabilities: a review of the literature', *Journal of Applied Research in Intellectual Disabilities*, 16: 1–9.

Whitehurst, T. (2006) 'Liberating silent voices: perspectives of children with profound and complex learning needs on inclusion', *British Journal of Learning Disabilities*, 35(1): 55–61.

Whittaker, A. (1997) *Looking at Our Services: Service Evaluation by People with Learning Difficulties*, London: King's Fund Centre.

Whittington, J. E., Butler, J. V., Holland, A. J. (2008) 'Pre-, peri- and postnatal complications in Prader–Willi syndrome in a UK sample', *Early Human Development*, 5: 331–6.

Wigham, S., Robertson, J., Emerson, E. *et al.* (2008) 'Reported goal setting and benefits of PCP for people with intellectual disabilities', *Journal of Intellectual Disabilities*, 12: 143–52.

Wightman, C. (2009) *Connecting People: The Steps to Making It Happen*, London: Foundation for People with Learning Disabilities.

Wilcox, E., Finlay, W. M. and Edmonds, J. (2006) '"His brain is totally different": An analysis of care–staff explanations of aggressive challenging behaviour and the impact of gendered discourses', *British Journal of Social Psychology*, 45: 197–216.

Wilkinson, H. and Janicki, M. (2002) 'The Edinburgh Principles with accompanying guidelines and recommendations', *Journal of Intellectual Disability Research*, 46(3): 279–84.

Williams, V. (1999) 'Researching together', *British Journal of Learning Disabilities*, 27(2): 48–51.

Williams, V. (2002) 'Being researchers with the label of Learning Difficulty: an analysis of talk in a project carried out by a self-advocacy research group', Ph.D. thesis, Milton Keynes, Open University.

Williams, V. (2011) *Disability and Discourse: Analysing Inclusive Conversation with People with Intellectual Disabilities*, Chichester: Wiley–Blackwell.

Williams, V. and Battleday, S. (2007) *Where do you want to go next? Critical Factors in Care Planning for People with Learning Disabilities, and Their Financial Implications*, Report for South West Regional Centre for Excellence.

Williams, V. and Heslop, P. (2005) 'Mental health support needs of people with a learning difficulty: a medical or a social model?', *Disability and Society*, 20(3): 231–46.

Williams, V. and Heslop, P. (2006) 'Filling the emotional gap at transition: young people with learning difficulties and friendship', *Tizard Learning Disability Review*, 11(4): 28–37.

Williams, V. and Holman, A. (2006) 'Direct payments and autonomy: issues for people with learning difficulties', in J. Leece and J. Bornat (eds), *Developments in Direct Payments*, Bristol: Policy Press, 65–78.

Williams, V. and Porter, S. (2011) *Your Life Your Choice: qualitative research as part of the Support Planning and Brokerage Initiative*, London: Office for Disability Issues.

Williams, V. and Robinson, C. (2000) *In Their Own Right: The Carers Act and Carers of People with Learning Disabilities*, Bristol: Policy Press.

Williams, V. and Robinson, C. (2001a) 'More than one wavelength: identifying, understanding and resolving conflicts of interest between people with intellectual disabilities and their family carers', *Journal of Applied Research in Intellectual Disabilities*, 14(1): 30–46.

Williams, V. and Robinson, C. (2001b) '"He'll finish up caring for me": people with learning disabilities and mutual support in the family', *British Journal of Learning Disabilities*, 29: 56–62.

Williams, V., Boyle, G., Jepson, M. *et al.* (2012) *Making Best Interests Decisions: People and Processes.* London: Mental Health Foundation, www.mhf.org.uk

Williams, V., Marriott, A. and Townsley, R. (2008a) *Shaping our Future: A Scoping and Consultation Exercise to Determine Research Priorities in Learning Disability for the Next Ten Years*, Report for the National Coordinating Centre for NHS Service Delivery and Organisation R&D (NCCSDO).

Williams, V., Jepson, M., Tarleton, B. and Marriott, A. (2008b) '"Listen to what I want": the potential implications of the Mental Capacity Act for major decision-making in adults with learning disabilities', London: Social Care Institute for Excellence.

Williams, V., Ponting, L., Ford, K. and Rudge, P. (2009a) '"A bit of common ground": personalisation and the use of shared knowledge in interactions between people with learning disabilities and their personal assistants', *Discourse Studies*, 11(5): 607–24.

Williams, V., Ponting, L., Ford, K. and Rudge, P. (2009b) '"I do like the subtle touch": interactions between people with learning disabilities and their personal assistants', *Disability and Society*, 24(7): 815–28.

Williams, V., Ponting, L., Ford, K. and Rudge, P. (2009c) 'Skills for support: personal assistants and people with learning disabilities', *British Journal of Learning Disabilities*, 38: 59–67.

Williams, V., Simons, K. and Swindon People First Research Team (2005) 'More researching together', *British Journal of Learning Disabilities*, 32: 1–9.

Williams, Victoria (2011) 'Talking about food: exploring attitudes towards food, health and obesity with adults with learning disabilities', Ph.D. thesis, University of Glasgow.

Williams, V., Boyle, G., Jepson, M. *et al.* (2012) *Making Best Interests Decisions: People and Processes*, London: Mental Health Foundation, www.mhf.org.uk

Windley, D. and Chapman, M. (2010) 'Support workers within learning/intellectual disability services perception of their role, training and support needs', *British Journal of Learning Disabilities*, 38: 310–18.

Winn, S. and Hay, I. (2009) 'Transition from school for youths with a disability: issues and challenges', *Disability and Society*, 24(1), 103–15.

Wistow, R. and Schneider, J. (2007) 'Employment support agencies in the UK: current operation and future development needs', *Health and Social Care in the Community*, 15: 128–35.

Wolfensberger, W. (1972) *The Principle of Normalization in Human Services*, Toronto: National Institution Mental Retardation.

Wooffitt, R. (2005) *Conversation Analysis and Discourse Analysis: A Comparative and Critical Introduction*, London: Sage.

Workman, A. (2008) 'People with a learning disability as home owners', *Llais*, winter, 2008/9: 3–6.

World Health Organization (2007) *Atlas: Global Resources for Person with Intellectual Disabilities*, Switzerland: World Health Organization.

Wright, A. M. (2006) 'Provision for students with learning difficulties in general colleges of further education – have we been going round in circles?', *British Journal of Special Education*, 33(1): 33–9.

Young, S. and Hawkins, T. (2006) 'Special parenting and the combined skills model', *Journal of Applied Research in Intellectual Disabilities*, 19: 346–55.

Index